Candida Overgrowth Treatment

Effective Dietary Strategies Recipes To Combat Candida And Build Immunity

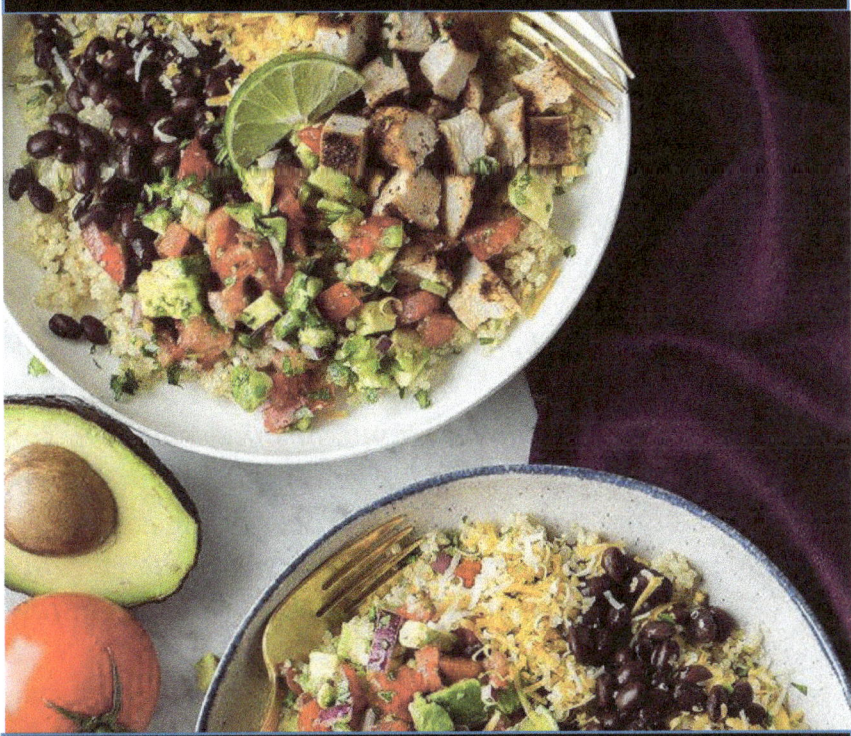

DR. WILFRED COLLINS

Copyright ©Wilfred Collins 2024. All rights reserved.

No part of this book may be reproduced, distributed, or transmitted in any form or by any means, including photocopying, recording, or other electronic or mechanical methods, without the prior written permission of the author, except in the case of brief quotations embodied in critical reviews and certain other noncommercial uses permitted by copyright law.

FOREWORD

Welcome to "Candida Overgrowth Treatment." This book is the culmination of my journey through understanding, managing, and ultimately thriving despite Candida overgrowth. Like many of you, I faced the myriad challenges that come with this often-overlooked condition—unexplained fatigue, persistent digestive issues, and the frustration of endless dietary restrictions. I embarked on a mission to regain control over my health, and what I discovered was transformative.

Candida overgrowth can affect anyone, and its impact on overall well-being is profound. As I navigated through the complexities of this condition, I realized that one of the most powerful tools for healing lies in the food we eat. This realization led me to explore the relationship between diet and Candida, resulting in the creation of this cookbook.

In "Candida Overgrowth Treatment," you will find more than just recipes; you will discover a comprehensive guide to understanding Candida, its causes, and its implications on health. I have included detailed information on how to recognize the symptoms, the importance of dietary choices, and practical tips for making lasting changes. Each chapter is designed to empower you with knowledge and practical tools to take control of your health.

The recipes in this book are crafted to be both delicious and nutritionally balanced. From the creamy Spinach and Avocado Soup to the vibrant Beet and Arugula Salad with Citrus Dressing, and the delightful Chia Seed Coconut Pudding, these dishes prove that eating Candida-friendly meals does not mean sacrificing flavor or enjoyment. Every recipe has been carefully selected to ensure it aligns with the principles of a Candida-friendly diet, making it easier for you to follow and enjoy.

This book is for anyone who has felt overwhelmed by the dietary changes necessary to manage Candida overgrowth. It's for those who are seeking not just to survive, but to thrive. It's for the home cooks, the busy professionals, the health enthusiasts, and everyone in between. My hope is that these recipes will bring you joy, comfort, and a sense of empowerment as you take charge of your health.

Thank you for allowing me to be a part of your journey. I am excited to share these recipes and insights with you, and I hope they will inspire you to embrace a healthier, more balanced lifestyle.

Here's to your health and happiness,

Dr. Wilfred Collins

ACKNOWLEDGEMENT

Writing this book has been an extraordinary odyssey, and I am profoundly appreciative of the myriad individuals whose support and encouragement have been pivotal to its fruition. Without their indispensable assistance, this book would not have come to life.

Primarily, I extend my most heartfelt thanks to my family and friends for their unwavering support and patience throughout this endeavor. Your belief in me has been a steadfast source of motivation and inspiration.

I am exceedingly grateful to my editor, whose astute eye and thoughtful feedback have significantly enhanced the caliber of this work. Your dedication to excellence and meticulous attention to detail have been instrumental in bringing this project to completion.

Special acknowledgment is due to the researchers and healthcare professionals who generously provided their expertise and insights on Candida overgrowth. Your contributions have enriched the content and ensured the accuracy and relevance of the information presented.

I would also like to express my gratitude to the recipe testers who enthusiastically engaged in trialing the dishes and offered invaluable feedback. Your efforts have been crucial in refining and perfecting the recipes, ensuring they are both delectable and practical for those adhering to a Candida-friendly diet.

A sincere thank you to my publisher for believing in this project and furnishing the resources and support necessary to bring it to life. Your guidance and professionalism have been immensely appreciated.

Lastly, I want to acknowledge the readers. Your interest in this book and your commitment to enhancing your health are what truly make this endeavor worthwhile. I hope that the knowledge and recipes shared within these pages will support you on your journey to better health and well-being.

Thank you all for being an integral part of this journey with me.

With deepest gratitude,

Dr. Wilfred Collins

TABLE OF CONTENT

FOREWORD 1

ACKNOWLEDGEMENT 5

INTRODUCTION: UNDERSTANDING CANDIDA . 10

Candida Overgrowth: Causes and Implications 10

The Role Of Diet In Managing Candida Overgrowth 14

Guidelines For Candida-Friendly Cooking 15

CHAPTER ONE: BREAKFAST DELIGHTS 18

ENERGIZING BREAKFAST SMOOTHIES 18

Berry Blast Smoothie 18

Green Power Smoothie 20

Coconut Almond Dream Smoothie 23

WHOLESOME BREAKFAST BOWLS 26

Quinoa Breakfast Bowl 26

Chia Seed Pudding with Fresh Berries 28

Vegetable Omelette With Herbs 31

CHAPTER TWO: NOURSHING SOUPS AND SALADS 34

HEALING VEGETABLE SOUPS 34

Butternut Squash And Ginger Soup 34

Creamy Cauliflower Soup 38

Spinach And Avocado Soup 40

FRESH AND FLAVORFUL SALADS 43

Kale And Quinoa Salad With Lemon Vinaigrette 43

Cucumber And Tomato Salad With Herbs 46

Beet And Arugula Salad With Citrus Dressing 48

CHAPTER THREE: SATISFYING MAIN DISHES . 52

PROTEIN-PACKED ENTREES 52

Baked Salmon With Lemon And Dill 52

Grilled Chicken With Herbed Quinoa 55

Lentil And Vegetable Stir-Fry 58

COMFORTING VEGETABLE DISHES 62

Roasted Garlic Brussels Sprouts 62

Zucchini Noodles With Pesto 65

Stuffed Bell Peppers With Brown Rice And Beans 68

CHAPTER FOUR: TASTY SNACKS AND DISHES 72

NUTRIENT-RICH SNACK IDEAS 72

Almond Butter And Apple Slices 72

Roasted Chickpeas With Spices 74

Raw Veggie Sticks With Hummus 77

FLAVORFUL SIDE DISHES 81

Garlic And Herb Quinoa 81

Steamed Broccoli With Lemon Butter Sauce 83

Mashed Cauliflower With Roasted Garlic 86
CHAPTER FIVE: SWEET TREATS AND DESSERTS 90
DECADENT DESSERT CREATIONS 90
Coconut Flour Banana Bread 90
Avocado Chocolate Mousse 93
Berry Coconut Ice Pops 96
INDULGENT SNACK IDEAS 99
Cacao Energy Balls 99
Baked Apple Chips With Cinnamon 101
Chia Seed Coconut Pudding 104
SUBSTITUTION GUIDE FOR CANDIDA-FRIENDLY INGREDIENTS 105
CONCLUSION 110

INTRODUCTION: UNDERSTANDING CANDIDA

- **Candida Overgrowth: Causes and Implications**

    Candida is a type of yeast or fungus that naturally exists in our body, typically in small amounts. It's commonly found on the skin, in the mouth, digestive tract, and genital area. While Candida is usually harmless, factors like a weakened immune system, certain medications, hormonal changes, and dietary habits can lead to its overgrowth. When Candida proliferates, it can cause infections such as oral thrush, genital yeast infections, and skin rashes. In severe cases, Candida can enter the bloodstream and cause systemic infections.

    Candida overgrowth occurs when there's an imbalance in the body's natural ecosystem, leading to an excessive proliferation of Candida yeast. Now, Candida is a normal part of our body's microbiota, which means it lives harmoniously with other microorganisms, especially in places like our mouth, gut, and genital areas. But sometimes, things can get out of balance.

There are several factors that can contribute to Candida overgrowth. Here are the key factors that can contribute to Candida overgrowth:

i. **Dietary Habits:** Consuming a diet high in sugar, refined carbohydrates, and processed foods provides an ideal environment for Candida to thrive. These foods can fuel the growth of yeast, leading to overgrowth.

ii. **Medications:** Certain medications, such as antibiotics, corticosteroids, and hormonal medications, can disrupt the balance of microorganisms in the body. Antibiotics, for example, can kill off beneficial bacteria that help keep Candida in check, allowing it to multiply unchecked.

iii. **Weakened Immune System:** A weakened immune system, whether due to stress, illness, or medical conditions like HIV/AIDS, can compromise the body's ability to regulate Candida levels. This makes individuals more susceptible to Candida overgrowth.

iv. **Hormonal Changes:** Hormonal fluctuations, such as those occurring during pregnancy, menstruation, or menopause, can alter the body's internal environment, potentially leading to Candida overgrowth.

v. **Underlying Health Conditions:** Certain underlying health conditions, such as diabetes, autoimmune disorders, and gastrointestinal disorders, can create an imbalance in the body's

microbiota, predisposing individuals to Candida overgrowth.
vi. **Poor Hygiene:** Inadequate hygiene practices, particularly in warm, moist areas of the body like the genital area or skin folds, can create conditions favorable for Candida growth.
vii. **Chronic Stress:** Chronic stress can weaken the immune system and disrupt the balance of microorganisms in the body, increasing the risk of Candida overgrowth.
viii. **Environmental Factors:** Environmental factors such as exposure to mold or damp environments can also contribute to Candida overgrowth, as these conditions can promote fungal growth.

Moreover, Candida overgrowth can have various implications for health and well-being, ranging from mild discomfort to serious complications. Here are some of the key implications:
i. **Localized Infections:** Candida overgrowth can lead to localized infections in areas such as the mouth (oral thrush), genital region (genital yeast infections), and skin (cutaneous candidiasis). These infections can cause symptoms such as itching, redness, soreness, and discharge, leading to discomfort and reduced quality of life.
ii. **Digestive Issues:** In some cases, Candida overgrowth in the digestive tract can contribute to digestive issues such as bloating, gas, diarrhea, or constipation. This can disrupt normal bowel

function and contribute to gastrointestinal discomfort.

iii. **Weakened Immune Response:** Chronic Candida overgrowth can tax the immune system, leading to a weakened immune response. This may increase susceptibility to other infections and illnesses, as the body's defenses are compromised.

iv. **Systemic Candidiasis:** In severe cases, Candida overgrowth can lead to systemic candidiasis, where the fungus enters the bloodstream and spreads throughout the body. Systemic candidiasis can cause symptoms such as fever, chills, fatigue, and muscle aches. If left untreated, it can lead to serious complications, including organ failure and sepsis.

v. **Chronic Health Conditions:** Some research suggests that chronic Candida overgrowth may be associated with certain chronic health conditions, such as autoimmune disorders, chronic fatigue syndrome, and fibromyalgia. While the exact relationship is still being studied, it's thought that Candida overgrowth may contribute to inflammation and immune dysregulation in these conditions.

vi. **Nutritional Deficiencies:** Candida overgrowth can interfere with nutrient absorption in the gut, potentially leading to nutritional deficiencies. This can further weaken the body's immune response and contribute to overall health issues.

vii. **Impact on Mental Health:** Some individuals with chronic Candida overgrowth may experience symptoms such as brain fog, mood swings, anxiety, or depression. While the exact mechanisms are not fully understood, it's believed that Candida overgrowth may contribute to these symptoms through its effects on gut health and inflammation.

■ The Role Of Diet In Managing Candida Overgrowth

Candida overgrowth, a condition characterized by the excessive proliferation of Candida yeast in the body, can be influenced by various factors, with diet playing a significant role in its management. While Candida is a normal part of the body's microbiota, an imbalance in the gut flora, often exacerbated by dietary habits, can lead to its overgrowth. Knowing the impact of diet on Candida and making appropriate dietary modifications is essential in managing this condition effectively.

The composition of one's diet can significantly influence the growth and proliferation of Candida yeast. Diets high in refined carbohydrates, sugars, and processed foods provide an abundant source of fuel for Candida, allowing it to multiply rapidly. These foods not only promote Candida growth but also disrupt the balance of beneficial bacteria in the gut, further exacerbating the overgrowth.

Conversely, a diet that is low in sugar and refined carbohydrates and rich in whole, nutrient-dense foods can help to create an environment in the body that is less conducive to Candida growth. High-fiber foods, such as fruits, vegetables, legumes, and whole grains, can support healthy digestion and promote the growth of beneficial bacteria in the gut, which can help to keep Candida in check.

■ Guidelines For Candida-Friendly Cooking

Let's take a look at some guildlines for Candida-friendly cooking:

1. **Limit Sugar and Refined Carbohydrates:** Avoid or minimize the use of sugar and refined carbohydrates in your cooking. Instead, opt for whole, unprocessed foods that are low in sugar and high in fiber. Choose complex carbohydrates such as whole grains, legumes, and non-starchy vegetables.
2. **Use Alternative Sweeteners:** When sweetening dishes, choose natural sweeteners that have minimal impact on blood sugar levels. Stevia, monk fruit extract, and erythritol are examples of low-calorie, natural sweeteners that can be used sparingly in Candida-friendly cooking.
3. **Incorporate Antifungal Ingredients:** Include ingredients with natural antifungal properties in your recipes to help combat Candida overgrowth. Garlic, onion, ginger, coconut oil, olive oil, and herbs like oregano, thyme, and rosemary are all excellent choices.

4. **Focus on Whole Foods:** Emphasize whole, nutrient-dense foods in your cooking, such as vegetables, fruits, lean proteins, nuts, seeds, and whole grains. These foods provide essential nutrients and fiber while minimizing the intake of substances that can promote Candida overgrowth.
5. **Opt for Fermented Foods:** Fermented foods are rich in probiotics, which are beneficial bacteria that can help restore balance to the gut microbiota and inhibit the growth of Candida. Include fermented foods such as yogurt, kefir, sauerkraut, kimchi, and kombucha in your diet.
6. **Choose Healthy Fats:** Incorporate healthy fats into your cooking, such as those found in avocados, nuts, seeds, olive oil, and coconut oil. These fats are important for supporting overall health and can help keep you feeling satisfied and full between meals.
7. **Experiment with Gluten-Free Grains:** While grains should be consumed in moderation on a Candida-friendly diet, gluten-free options such as quinoa, brown rice, millet, and buckwheat can be enjoyed occasionally. These grains are less likely to contribute to Candida overgrowth compared to their gluten-containing counterparts.
8. **Hydrate with Water:** Stay hydrated by drinking plenty of water throughout the day. Water helps flush toxins from the body and supports optimal digestion, which is important for maintaining a healthy balance of microorganisms in the gut.

9. **Be Mindful of Food Combining:** Pay attention to how you combine foods in your recipes. Some food combinations can be more difficult to digest and may exacerbate digestive issues. Try to keep meals balanced and include a variety of foods to support optimal digestion.
10. **Listen to Your Body:** Finally, listen to your body and pay attention to how different foods make you feel. Everyone's dietary needs are unique, so it's important to experiment and find what works best for you. If certain foods trigger symptoms of Candida overgrowth, consider eliminating or reducing them from your diet.

CHAPTER ONE
BREAKFAST DELIGHTS

ENERGIZING BREAKFAST SMOOTHIES

■ Berry Blast Smoothie

The Berry Blast Smoothie is a beverage that's perfect for supporting your health while managing Candida overgrowth. Bursting with the goodness of antioxidant-rich berries and probiotic-containing yogurt, this smoothie is not only delicious but also offers a host of health benefits.

Ingredients:
i. A handful of mixed berries (strawberries, blueberries, raspberries, blackberries)
ii. Plain yogurt or kefir
iii. Leafy greens (optional, for an extra nutrient boost)
iv. Liquid base (water, coconut water, almond milk, or coconut milk)

v. Optional boosters (chia seeds, flaxseeds, protein powder, nut butter)

Cooking Methods:
- **Preparation:** Wash the berries and leafy greens thoroughly. If using leafy greens, remove any tough stems.
- **Assembly:** In a blender, combine the mixed berries, yogurt or kefir, leafy greens (if using), and liquid base of your choice.
- **Optional Additions:** Add any optional boosters such as chia seeds, flaxseeds, protein powder, or nut butter for additional nutrients and texture.
- **Blend:** Blend all the ingredients until smooth and creamy. If the consistency is too thick, add more liquid until desired consistency is reached.
- **Taste Test:** Taste the smoothie and adjust sweetness or tanginess as desired by adding a touch of honey or lemon juice.

The Berry Blast Smoothie comes together quickly, requiring just 5 minutes for preparation and an additional 1 to 2 minutes for blending. Each serving packs a nutritional punch, providing approximately 150-200 calories, though this may vary depending on the specific ingredients and any optional additions. Rich in antioxidants, vitamins, minerals, probiotics, and fiber, this smoothie offers a nourishing boost to support overall health and well-being. With a recommended serving size of one smoothie per person, it's a satisfying and guilt-free treat that fits perfectly into a Candida-friendly diet.

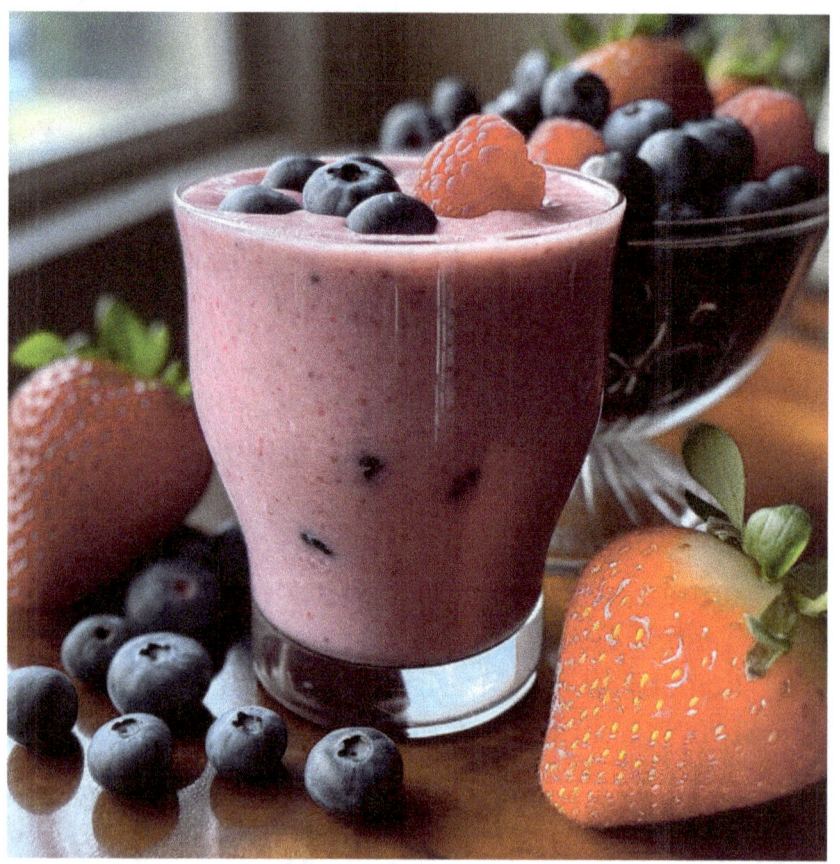

Berry Blast Smoothie

■ Green Power Smoothie

The Green Power Smoothie is a vibrant and nutrient-packed beverage that provides a refreshing burst of energy and vitality. This invigorating smoothie combines an array of green vegetables and fruits, along with other nutritious ingredients, to create a delicious and satisfying drink that supports overall health and well-being. Packed with vitamins, minerals, fiber, and antioxidants, this smoothie is a perfect addition to your Candida-friendly diet.

Ingredients:
i. 1 cup spinach leaves
ii. 1/2 cup kale leaves, stemmed
iii. 1/2 cucumber, chopped
iv. 1/2 green apple, cored and chopped
v. 1/2 avocado, pitted and peeled
vi. 1/2 lemon, juiced
vii. 1 tablespoon fresh ginger, grated
viii. 1 cup coconut water or water
ix. Optional: a handful of fresh mint leaves or parsley for added freshness

Cooking Methods:
- **Preparation:** Wash the spinach, kale, cucumber, apple, and ginger thoroughly under running water. Remove any tough stems from the spinach and kale. Core and chop the apple, peel and pit the avocado, and juice the lemon.
- **Blending:** In a blender, combine the spinach, kale, cucumber, apple, avocado, ginger, and lemon juice. Add the coconut water or water to help facilitate blending.
- **Blend Until Smooth:** Blend all the ingredients until smooth and creamy. You may need to stop and scrape down the sides of the blender

occasionally to ensure everything is well incorporated.
- ➢ **Adjust Consistency**: If the smoothie is too thick, you can add more liquid (coconut water or water) to achieve the desired consistency. Conversely, if it's too thin, you can add more greens or avocado to thicken it up.
- ➢ **Optional**: For an extra burst of freshness, you can add a handful of fresh mint leaves or parsley to the blender and blend until finely chopped and incorporated into the smoothie.

The Green Power Smoothie is quick and easy to prepare, with a total cooking time of just 5 minutes per serving. From washing and chopping the ingredients to blending them together, you'll have a delicious and nutritious smoothie ready to enjoy in no time. So, whether you're starting your day with a boost of energy or refueling after a workout, the Green Power Smoothie is the perfect choice for a healthy and satisfying drink.

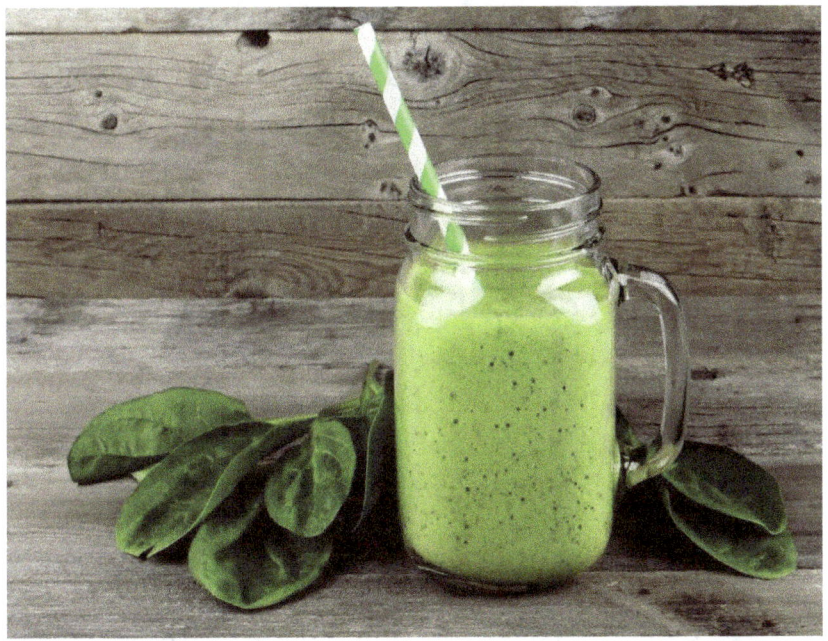

■ Coconut Almond Dream Smoothie

The Coconut Almond Dream Smoothie is a creamy and satisfying beverage that offers a delightful blend of tropical flavors and nutritious ingredients. Perfect for breakfast or as a refreshing snack, this smoothie will transport you to a tropical paradise with every sip.

Ingredients:
To make the Coconut Almond Dream Smoothie, you'll need the following ingredients:
i. 1 ripe banana, peeled and sliced
ii. 1/2 cup unsweetened coconut milk
iii. 1/4 cup plain Greek yogurt

iv. 2 tablespoons almond butter
v. 1 tablespoon unsweetened shredded coconut
vi. 1/4 teaspoon vanilla extract
vii. Ice cubes (optional, for a colder smoothie)

Cooking Method:
- Start by adding the sliced banana, coconut milk, Greek yogurt, almond butter, shredded coconut, and vanilla extract to a blender.
- If desired, add a handful of ice cubes for a colder and more refreshing smoothie.
- Blend all the ingredients until smooth and creamy, scraping down the sides of the blender as needed to ensure everything is well combined.
- Once the smoothie reaches your desired consistency, pour it into a glass and garnish with a sprinkle of shredded coconut, if desired.

The Coconut Almond Dream Smoothie comes together in just a few minutes, making it a quick and convenient option for busy mornings or whenever you need a nutritious pick-me-up. Each serving of this smoothie provides a generous dose of healthy fats from the almond butter and coconut, along with protein from the Greek yogurt. It's a delicious and satisfying way to start your day or refuel after a workout. Plus, with its tropical flavors and creamy texture, it's sure to become a favorite in your Candida-friendly recipe repertoire.

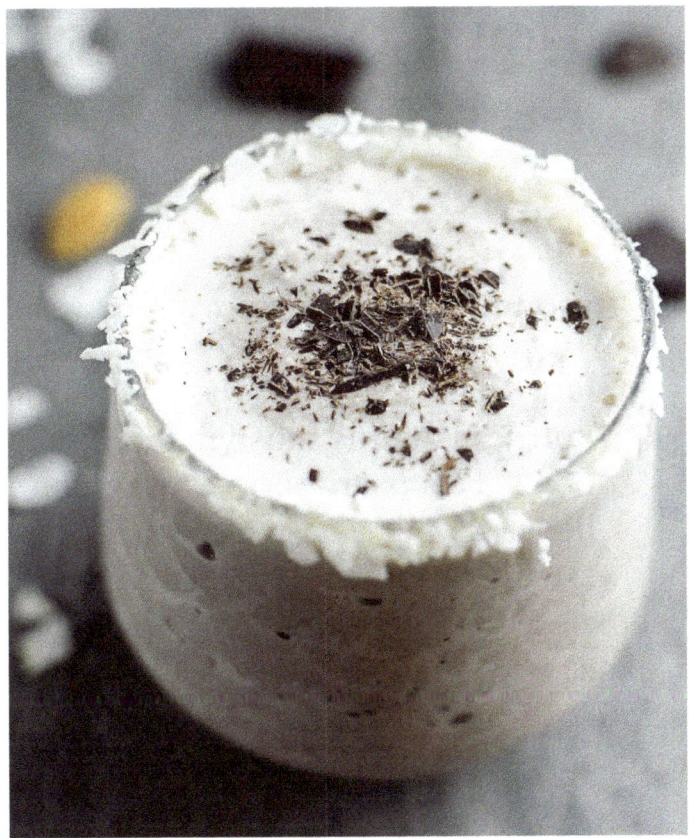

Coconut Almond Dream Smoothie

WHOLESOME BREAKFAST BOWLS

■ Quinoa Breakfast Bowl

Start your day on the right foot with a nutritious and satisfying Quinoa Breakfast Bowl. This hearty breakfast option is not only delicious but also packed with protein, fiber, and essential nutrients to fuel your morning. Whether you're looking for a quick and easy breakfast or a leisurely weekend brunch, this versatile dish is sure to please your taste buds and keep you feeling satisfied until lunchtime.

Ingredients:
For your Quinoa Breakfast Bowl, you'll need:
i. 1/2 cup quinoa
ii. 1 cup water or milk of your choice
iii. Your favorite toppings such as fresh fruit (berries, banana slices), nuts (almonds, walnuts), seeds (chia seeds, pumpkin seeds), dried fruit (raisins, cranberries), honey or maple syrup, and a sprinkle of cinnamon or nutmeg for extra flavor.

Cooking Method:
➢ Rinse the quinoa under cold water to remove any bitterness.

- In a small saucepan, combine the rinsed quinoa and water or milk. Bring to a boil over medium-high heat.
- Once boiling, reduce the heat to low, cover, and simmer for about 15 minutes, or until the quinoa is tender and has absorbed all the liquid. You'll know it's ready when you see little spirals (germ rings) separating from and curling around the quinoa seeds.
- Remove the saucepan from the heat and let it sit, covered, for 5 minutes to allow the quinoa to steam and fluff up.
- Fluff the quinoa with a fork and transfer it to a bowl.
- Top your cooked quinoa with your favorite toppings, such as fresh fruit, nuts, seeds, dried fruit, honey or maple syrup, and a sprinkle of cinnamon or nutmeg.

This Quinoa Breakfast Bowl takes about 20 minutes to prepare, from start to finish, making it perfect for busy mornings. It serves one generously, but you can easily double or triple the recipe to feed a crowd or meal prep for the week ahead. Each serving is packed with protein, fiber, and essential nutrients, providing a nutritious and satisfying start to your day.

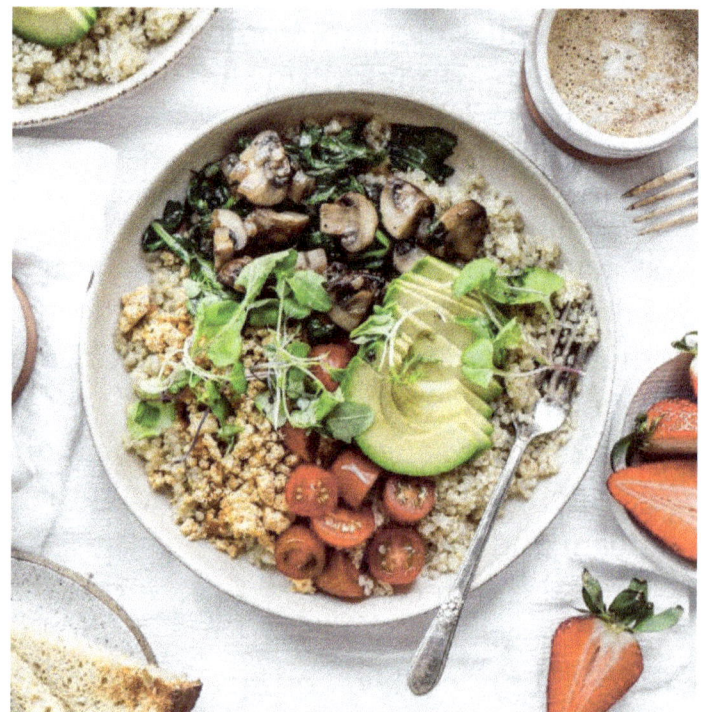

Quinoa Breakfast Bowl

■ Chia Seed Pudding with Fresh Berries

Chia Seed Pudding with Fresh Berries is a delightful dessert option that is not only delicious but also perfect for those following a Candida-friendly diet. This creamy pudding is made with chia seeds, which are rich in fiber, omega-3 fatty acids, and antioxidants, and topped with fresh berries, adding a burst of flavor and additional nutritional benefits.

Ingredients:

To make Chia Seed Pudding with Fresh Berries, you will need:

i. 1/4 cup chia seeds
ii. 1 cup unsweetened almond milk (or any other dairy-free milk of your choice)
iii. 1 tablespoon pure maple syrup or honey (optional, adjust to taste)
iv. 1/2 teaspoon vanilla extract
v. Fresh berries of your choice (such as strawberries, blueberries, raspberries) for topping

Cooking Methods:

- In a mixing bowl or jar, combine the chia seeds, almond milk, maple syrup or honey (if using), and vanilla extract. Stir well to ensure that the chia seeds are evenly distributed and no clumps remain.
- Cover the bowl or jar and refrigerate the mixture for at least 2 hours, or preferably overnight. During this time, the chia seeds will absorb the liquid and swell, resulting in a thick and creamy pudding-like consistency.
- Once the chia seed pudding has set, give it a good stir to break up any clumps and ensure a smooth texture. If the pudding is too thick, you can add a splash of almond milk to reach your desired consistency.
- To serve, divide the chia seed pudding into individual bowls or jars and top with a generous portion of fresh berries. You can use a mix of strawberries, blueberries, raspberries, or any other berries you prefer.

Chia Seed Pudding with Fresh Berries is incredibly easy to make and requires minimal hands-on cooking time. The majority of the time is spent waiting for the pudding to set in the refrigerator, which typically takes around 2 hours but can be left overnight for convenience. This recipe makes approximately 2 servings, depending on portion size. Each serving of Chia Seed Pudding with Fresh Berries is a nutritious and satisfying treat that is low in sugar and high in fiber, antioxidants, and omega-3 fatty acids. It's the perfect guilt-free dessert option for those looking to indulge their sweet tooth while nourishing their body with wholesome ingredients.

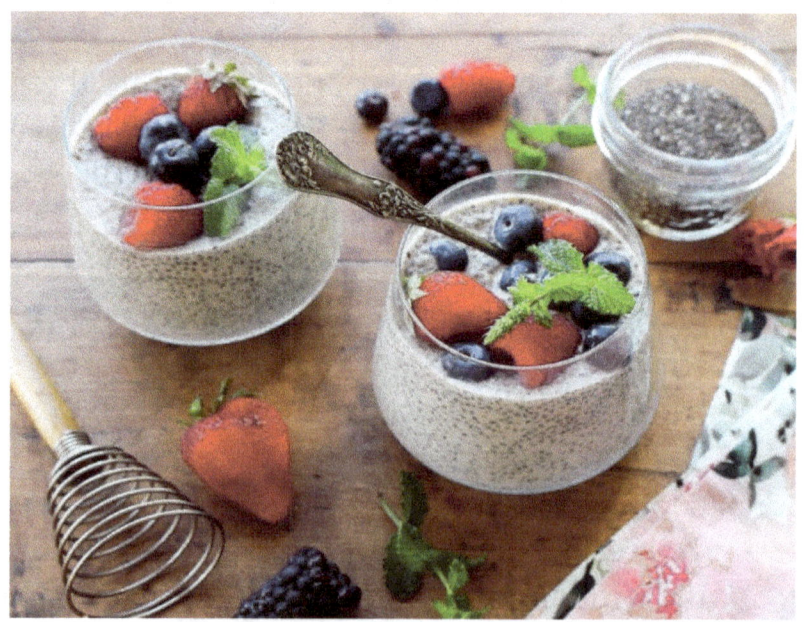

Chia Seeds Pudding With Fresh Berries

■ Vegetable Omelette With Herbs

A Vegetable Omelette with Herbs is a versatile and nutritious dish that can be enjoyed for breakfast, brunch, or even a light dinner. This satisfying meal combines fluffy eggs with a colorful array of vegetables and fragrant herbs, resulting in a flavorful and wholesome dish that is both easy to prepare and incredibly satisfying.

Ingredients:
To make a Vegetable Omelette with Herbs, you will need:
i. Eggs: 2-3 large eggs per serving
ii. Assorted Vegetables: such as bell peppers, onions, tomatoes, spinach, mushrooms, or any other vegetables of your choice, finely chopped
iii. Fresh Herbs: such as parsley, cilantro, basil, or dill, finely chopped
iv. Salt and Pepper: to taste
v. Olive Oil or Butter: for cooking

Cooking Method:
- **Prepare the Vegetables:** Heat a tablespoon of olive oil or butter in a non-stick skillet over medium heat. Add the chopped vegetables of your choice and sauté until they are tender and lightly caramelized, about 5-7 minutes. Season with salt and pepper to taste.
- **Whisk the Eggs:** While the vegetables are cooking, crack the eggs into a bowl and whisk them

together until well combined. Season with salt and pepper to taste. Stir in the chopped fresh herbs.
- ➤ **Cook the Omelette:** Once the vegetables are cooked, spread them evenly across the skillet in a single layer. Pour the whisked eggs over the vegetables, ensuring that they are evenly distributed. Allow the omelette to cook undisturbed for 2-3 minutes, or until the edges begin to set.
- ➤ **Fold and Finish:** Using a spatula, gently lift the edges of the omelette and fold them towards the center. Continue cooking for another 2-3 minutes, or until the eggs are fully set and the omelette is golden brown on the bottom.
- ➤ **Serve:** Once the omelette is cooked to your liking, carefully slide it onto a plate and garnish with additional fresh herbs, if desired. Cut the omelette into wedges and serve hot, accompanied by your favorite sides such as whole-grain toast, salad, or roasted potatoes.

The cooking time for a Vegetable Omelette with Herbs will vary depending on the thickness of the omelette and the heat of your stove. Generally, it takes about 10-15 minutes to prepare and cook the omelette from start to finish.

Per serving, this Vegetable Omelette with Herbs is a satisfying and nutritious meal that provides a balanced combination of protein, vitamins, and fiber. It's a perfect option for a quick and healthy breakfast or brunch, and can be customized with your favorite vegetables and herbs to suit your taste preferences. Enjoy this flavorful omelette as a delicious and nourishing addition to your Candida-friendly diet.

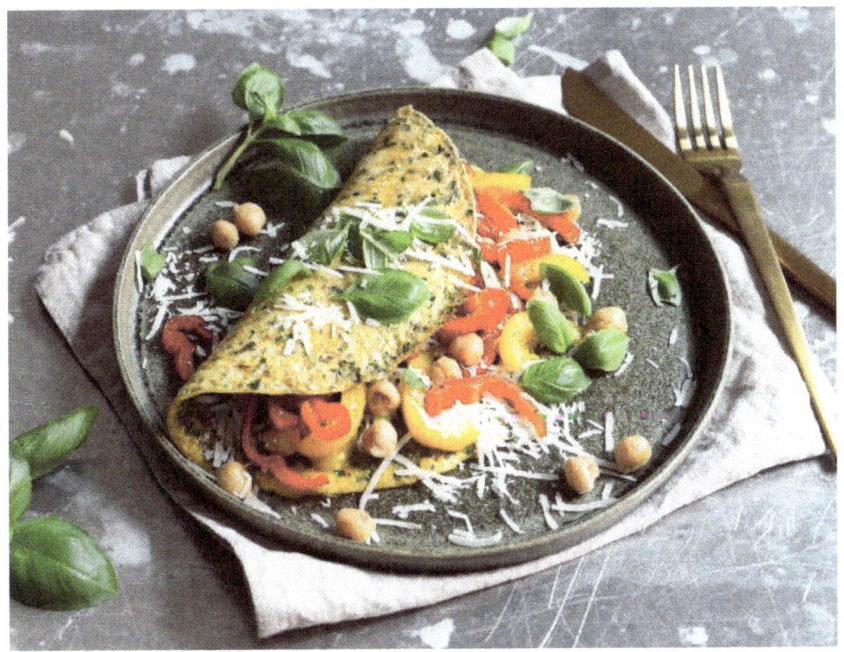

Vegetabel Omelette With Herbs

CHAPTER TWO
NOURSHING SOUPS AND SALADS

HEALING VEGETABLE SOUPS

■ Butternut Squash And Ginger Soup

Warm, comforting, and bursting with flavor, Butternut Squash and Ginger Soup is a delightful dish that soothes the soul and nourishes the body. This creamy soup combines the natural sweetness of butternut squash with the subtle heat of ginger, creating a perfect harmony of flavors. Whether enjoyed as a light lunch or a cozy dinner option, this soup is sure to become a favorite in your Candida-friendly kitchen.

Ingredients:
i. 1 medium butternut squash, peeled, seeded, and diced
ii. 1 tablespoon olive oil
iii. 1 onion, chopped

iv. 2 cloves garlic, minced
v. 1 tablespoon fresh ginger, grated
vi. 4 cups vegetable broth
vii. Salt and pepper, to taste
viii. Optional toppings: toasted pumpkin seeds, a drizzle of coconut cream, or chopped fresh herbs

Cooking Methods:
- **Preparation:** Begin by peeling, seeding, and dicing the butternut squash. Chop the onion, mince the garlic, and grate the fresh ginger.
- **Sauté Aromatics:** In a large pot, heat the olive oil over medium heat. Add the chopped onion and sauté until softened, about 5 minutes. Add the minced garlic and grated ginger, and cook for an additional 1-2 minutes until fragrant.
- **Add Squash:** Add the diced butternut squash to the pot, along with the vegetable broth. Bring the mixture to a boil, then reduce the heat to low, cover, and simmer for 20-25 minutes, or until the squash is tender and easily pierced with a fork.
- **Blend Soup:** Once the squash is cooked, use an immersion blender to purée the soup until smooth and creamy. Alternatively, transfer the soup in batches to a blender and blend until smooth. Season the soup with salt and pepper to taste, adjusting the seasoning as needed.
- **Serve:** Ladle the Butternut Squash and Ginger Soup into bowls and garnish with optional toppings such as toasted pumpkin seeds, a drizzle

of coconut cream, or chopped fresh herbs. Serve hot and enjoy!

This Butternut Squash and Ginger Soup comes together in just under 45 minutes, making it a quick and convenient option for a wholesome meal. With its creamy texture and rich flavors, it's perfect for warming up on chilly days or enjoying as a light and nourishing meal any time of year. This recipe makes approximately 4 servings, so it's great for sharing with family and friends or for enjoying as leftovers throughout the week. Each serving is a comforting bowl of goodness, providing a generous dose of vitamins, minerals, and fiber to support your health and well-being.

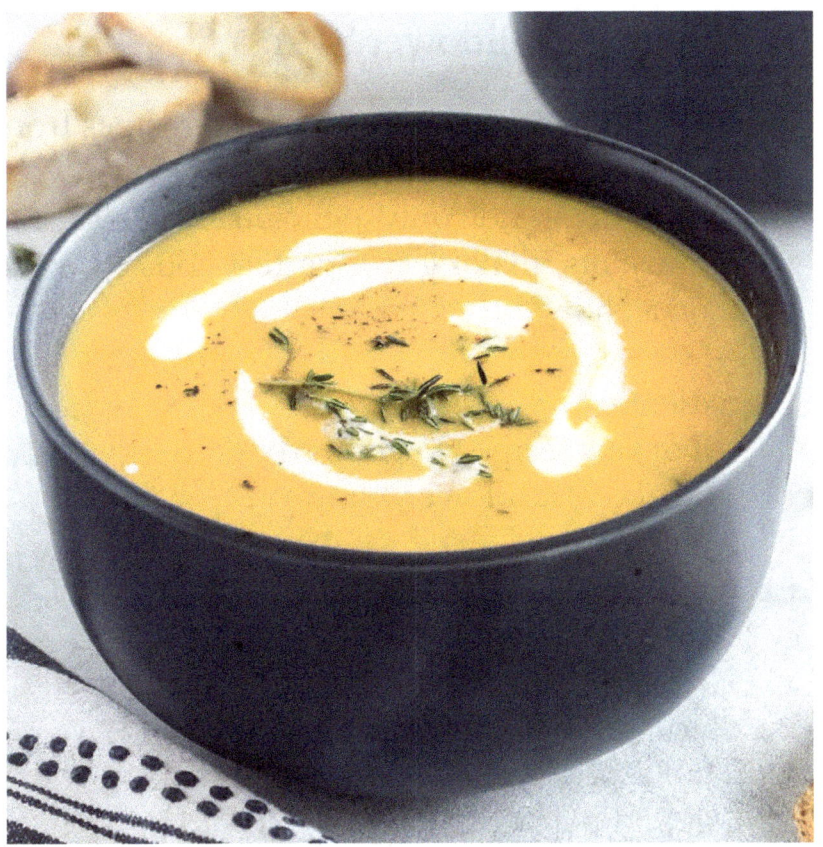

Butternut Squash And Ginger Soup

■ Creamy Cauliflower Soup

Introducing one of our favorite recipes from the book: Creamy Cauliflower Soup! This velvety-smooth soup is not only delicious but also packed with nutrients, making it a perfect choice for a cozy meal on a chilly day.

Ingredients:
For this recipe, you'll need:
i. 1 head of cauliflower, chopped
ii. 1 onion, diced
iii. 2 cloves of garlic, minced
iv. 4 cups of vegetable broth
v. 1 cup of unsweetened almond milk (or any non-dairy milk of your choice)
vi. 2 tablespoons of olive oil
vii. Salt and pepper to taste
viii. Optional garnishes: chopped chives, crispy bacon bits, or a drizzle of olive oil

Cooking Method:
- **Sauté the Aromatics:** In a large pot, heat olive oil over medium heat. Add diced onion and minced garlic, and sauté until soft and fragrant, about 5 minutes.
- **Add the Cauliflower:** Add the chopped cauliflower to the pot, and stir to combine with the onions and garlic.
- **Simmer:** Pour in the vegetable broth, and bring the mixture to a simmer. Cover the pot and let it

simmer for about 20-25 minutes, or until the cauliflower is tender and easily pierced with a fork.
- **Blend:** Once the cauliflower is cooked, use an immersion blender to puree the soup until smooth and creamy. Alternatively, you can transfer the soup to a blender in batches and blend until smooth.
- **Add the Almond Milk:** Stir in the almond milk to achieve your desired consistency. If the soup is too thick, you can add more almond milk or vegetable broth until you reach the desired thickness.
- **Season:** Season the soup with salt and pepper to taste, adjusting as needed.
- **Serve:** Ladle the creamy cauliflower soup into bowls and garnish with chopped chives, crispy bacon bits, or a drizzle of olive oil, if desired.

This Creamy Cauliflower Soup takes about 30-35 minutes to prepare from start to finish, making it a quick and easy option for a weeknight dinner. Plus, it yields about 4 servings, so you can enjoy it as a satisfying meal for the whole family or save leftovers for lunch the next day. With its creamy texture, comforting flavor, and nutrient-rich ingredients, our Creamy Cauliflower Soup is sure to become a staple in your kitchen. So, grab a spoon and cozy up with a bowl of this delicious soup – you won't be disappointed!

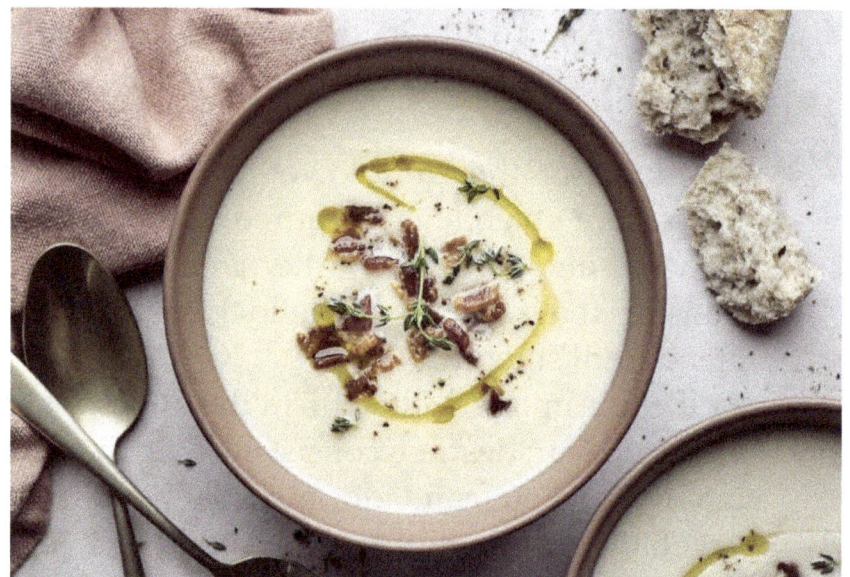

Creamy Cauliflower Soup

■ Spinach And Avocado Soup

Indulge in the creamy goodness of Spinach and Avocado Soup, a nourishing and flavorful dish that combines the vibrant green hues of spinach with the velvety texture of ripe avocados. This soup is not only delicious but also packed with nutrients, making it a perfect choice for those seeking a wholesome and satisfying meal on their Candida-friendly journey.

Ingredients:

For this delightful soup, you'll need:

i. Fresh spinach leaves: 4 cups, washed and chopped
ii. Ripe avocados: 2, peeled and diced

iii. Vegetable broth: 4 cups
iv. Onion: 1 medium, chopped
v. Garlic cloves: 2, minced
vi. Olive oil: 2 tablespoons
vii. Lemon juice: 2 tablespoons
viii. Salt and pepper: to taste

Cooking Methods:

- **Sauté Aromatics:** In a large pot, heat olive oil over medium heat. Add chopped onion and minced garlic, and sauté until fragrant and translucent, about 3-4 minutes.
- **Add Spinach:** Add the chopped spinach leaves to the pot, stirring occasionally until wilted, about 2-3 minutes.
- **Blend:** Transfer the sautéed spinach mixture to a blender or food processor. Add diced avocados, vegetable broth, and lemon juice. Blend until smooth and creamy, adjusting the consistency with additional vegetable broth if desired.
- **Season:** Season the soup with salt and pepper to taste, adjusting as needed to suit your preferences.
- **Serve:** Ladle the Spinach and Avocado Soup into bowls and garnish with a drizzle of olive oil, a sprinkle of freshly ground black pepper, or a wedge of lemon for an extra burst of flavor.

This Spinach and Avocado Soup comes together in just under 20 minutes, making it a quick and convenient option for busy weeknights or lazy weekends. With its creamy texture and vibrant green color, it's sure to impress both your taste buds and your guests. Plus, each serving is a nutrient-rich delight, providing a generous dose of vitamins, minerals, and healthy fats to nourish your body and support your Candida-friendly lifestyle. So go ahead, dig in, and savor every spoonful of this delectable soup!

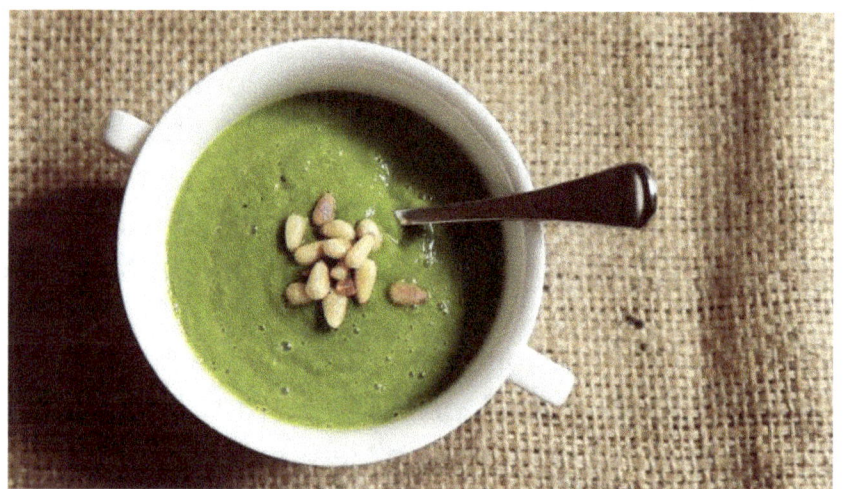

Spinach And Avocado Soup

FRESH AND FLAVORFUL SALADS

■ Kale And Quinoa Salad With Lemon Vinaigrette

Kale and Quinoa Salad with Lemon Vinaigrette is a vibrant, nutritious dish that brings together the hearty, nutrient-dense qualities of kale and quinoa, paired with a refreshing lemon vinaigrette. This salad is perfect for those looking to maintain a healthy, balanced diet while managing Candida overgrowth. It's not only delicious but also packed with vitamins, minerals, and protein, making it a satisfying meal or side dish.

Ingredients:
For this wholesome salad, you will need:
i. Kale: 6 cups, washed and chopped
ii. Quinoa: 1 cup, rinsed
iii. Water: 2 cups (for cooking quinoa)
iv. Cherry tomatoes: 1 cup, halved
v. Cucumber: 1 medium, diced
vi. Red bell pepper: 1, diced
vii. Red onion: 1/2, finely chopped
viii. Feta cheese (optional): 1/2 cup, crumbled
ix. Slivered almonds: 1/4 cup, toasted

For the Lemon Vinaigrette:
i. Fresh lemon juice: 1/4 cup
ii. Olive oil: 1/3 cup
iii. Dijon mustard: 1 teaspoon
iv. Honey or a Candida-friendly sweetener: 1 teaspoon
v. Garlic: 1 clove, minced
vi. Salt and pepper: to taste

Cooking Methods:
- **Cook the Quinoa:** In a medium saucepan, bring 2 cups of water to a boil. Add the rinsed quinoa, reduce the heat to low, cover, and simmer for about 15 minutes or until the quinoa is cooked and the water is absorbed. Fluff with a fork and set aside to cool.
- **Prepare the Kale:** While the quinoa is cooking, place the chopped kale in a large mixing bowl. Massage the kale with a small amount of olive oil and a pinch of salt for about 2-3 minutes. This helps to soften the kale and make it more palatable.
- **Chop the Vegetables:** Prepare the cherry tomatoes, cucumber, red bell pepper, and red onion by chopping them into bite-sized pieces. Add these vegetables to the bowl with the kale.
- **Make the Vinaigrette:** In a small bowl or jar, whisk together the lemon juice, olive oil, Dijon mustard, honey, minced garlic, salt, and pepper until well combined.

➢ **Assemble the Salad:** Add the cooled quinoa to the bowl with the kale and vegetables. Pour the lemon vinaigrette over the salad and toss everything together until well coated. If using, sprinkle the crumbled feta cheese and toasted slivered almonds on top.

This Kale and Quinoa Salad with Lemon Vinaigrette can be prepared in about 30 minutes, making it a quick and nutritious option for any meal. Each serving is packed with protein, fiber, and essential nutrients, providing a balanced and satisfying dish that's perfect for lunch, dinner, or as a side. The tangy lemon vinaigrette adds a refreshing zing, complementing the robust flavors of the kale and quinoa. Enjoy this salad fresh, or store it in the refrigerator for a convenient, healthy meal prep option.

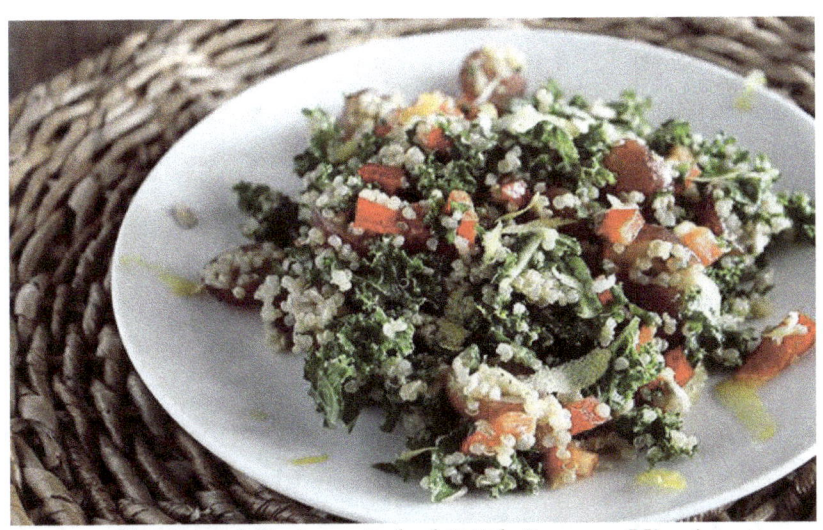

Kale And Quinoa Salad With Lemon Vinaigrette

■ Cucumber And Tomato Salad With Herbs

The Cucumber and Tomato Salad with Herbs is a refreshing dish that celebrates the natural flavors of fresh vegetables. This salad is not only simple to prepare but also incredibly nutritious, making it an ideal choice for a Candida-friendly diet. Packed with crisp cucumbers, juicy tomatoes, and aromatic herbs, this salad is a perfect accompaniment to any meal or a light, satisfying snack on its own.

Ingredients:
To make this delightful salad, you'll need:
i. Cucumbers: 2 medium, peeled and thinly sliced
ii. Tomatoes: 3 medium, diced
iii. Red onion: 1 small, thinly sliced
iv. Fresh parsley: 1/4 cup, chopped
v. Fresh basil: 1/4 cup, chopped
vi. Olive oil: 3 tablespoons
vii. Lemon juice: 2 tablespoons
viii. Salt: to taste
ix. Black pepper: to taste

Cooking Methods:
➢ **Prepare Vegetables:** Start by preparing the vegetables. Peel and thinly slice the cucumbers, dice the tomatoes, and thinly slice the red onion. Place them in a large mixing bowl.

- ➢ **Chop Herbs:** Chop the fresh parsley and basil finely and add them to the bowl with the vegetables. The fresh herbs add a burst of flavor and fragrance to the salad.
- ➢ **Dress the Salad:** In a small bowl, whisk together the olive oil and lemon juice to make a simple and light dressing. Pour this dressing over the vegetables and herbs in the mixing bowl.
- ➢ **Toss and Season:** Gently toss all the ingredients together to ensure they are well combined and evenly coated with the dressing. Season the salad with salt and black pepper to taste, adjusting the seasoning according to your preference.
- ➢ **Serve:** Transfer the Cucumber and Tomato Salad with Herbs to a serving dish. For an added touch, you can garnish it with a few extra sprigs of fresh herbs or a lemon wedge on the side.

This Cucumber and Tomato Salad with Herbs is quick and easy to prepare, taking only about 15 minutes from start to finish. It's a perfect option for a quick lunch, a refreshing side dish for dinner, or a light snack. Each serving is packed with fresh, wholesome ingredients that are both delicious and beneficial for maintaining a balanced diet. Enjoy the crisp textures and vibrant flavors of this salad, knowing it's a nutritious choice for your Candida-friendly lifestyle.

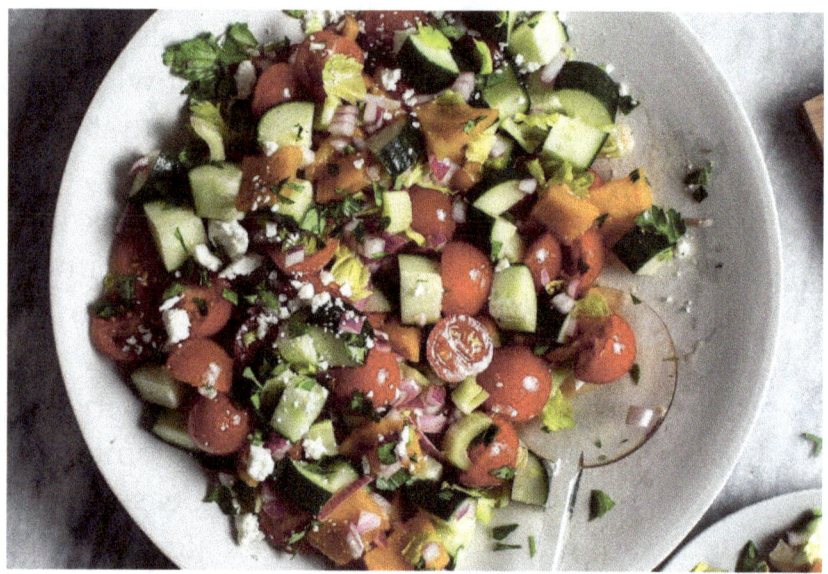

Cucmber And Tomato Salad With Herbs

■ Beet And Arugula Salad With Citrus Dressing

The Beet and Arugula Salad with Citrus Dressing is a vibrant and comforting dish that combines the earthy sweetness of beets with the peppery bite of arugula, all brought together by a tangy citrus dressing. This salad is not only visually appealing but also packed with nutrients, making it a perfect addition to a Candida-friendly diet. Whether you're looking for a light lunch or a side dish, this salad is sure to delight your taste buds and nourish your body.

Ingredients:

For the Beet and Arugula Salad, you will need:

i. Beets: 4 medium-sized, cooked and sliced
ii. Arugula: 4 cups, washed and dried
iii. Orange: 1, peeled and segmented
iv. Goat cheese: 1/2 cup, crumbled (optional for extra creaminess)
v. Walnuts: 1/4 cup, toasted

For the Citrus Dressing:
i. Orange juice: 1/4 cup, freshly squeezed
ii. Lemon juice: 2 tablespoons, freshly squeezed
iii. Olive oil: 1/4 cup
iv. Dijon mustard: 1 teaspoon
v. Honey or stevia: 1 teaspoon (optional for a hint of sweetness)
vi. Salt and pepper: to taste

Cooking Methods:
- **Prepare the Beets:** If not already cooked, boil or roast the beets until tender. To boil, place beets in a pot of water and cook for about 30-40 minutes until they can be easily pierced with a fork. For roasting, wrap beets in aluminum foil and bake at 400°F (200°C) for about 45-60 minutes. Once cooked, allow them to cool, then peel and slice them into thin rounds or wedges.
- **Make the Dressing:** In a small bowl, whisk together the freshly squeezed orange juice, lemon juice, olive oil, Dijon mustard, and honey or stevia (if using). Season with salt and pepper to taste, adjusting the flavors as needed.

- **Assemble the Salad:** In a large salad bowl, combine the arugula, cooked and sliced beets, orange segments, and toasted walnuts. If using, sprinkle the crumbled goat cheese over the top.
- **Dress the Salad:** Drizzle the citrus dressing over the salad just before serving. Toss gently to ensure all the ingredients are evenly coated with the dressing.

This Beet and Arugula Salad with Citrus Dressing can be prepared in about 20-30 minutes, depending on whether you need to cook the beets. It's a quick and easy dish that serves approximately four people, making it a great choice for a family meal or a small gathering. The combination of flavors and textures in this salad – from the sweet, tender beets to the crisp, peppery arugula and the creamy goat cheese – creates a delightful and nutritious dish that is sure to please. Enjoy this salad as a light lunch, a refreshing side dish, or a beautiful starter for your Candida-friendly menu.

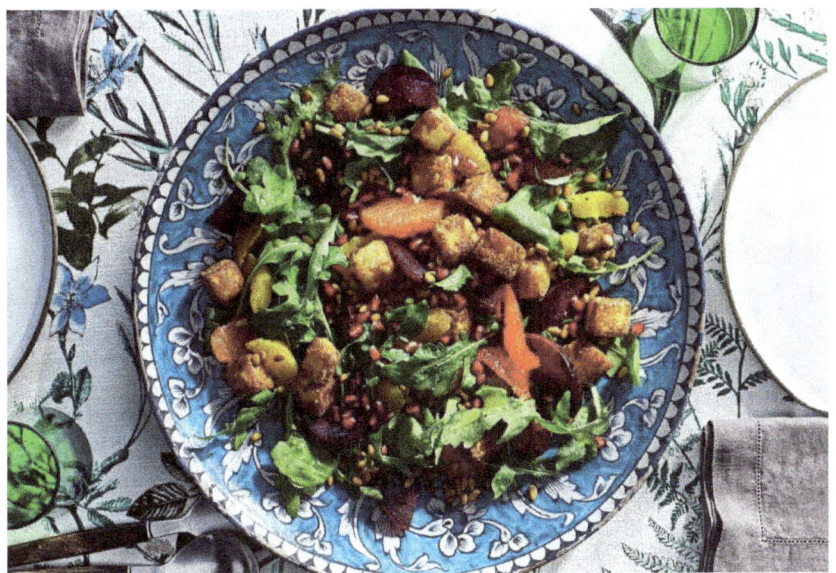

Beet And Arugula Salad With Citrus Dressing

CHAPTER THREE
SATISFYING MAIN DISHES

PROTEIN-PACKED ENTREES

■ Baked Salmon With Lemon And Dill

Baked Salmon with Lemon and Dill showcases the rich flavors of salmon enhanced by the fresh, zesty taste of lemon and the aromatic notes of dill. This dish falls into the protein class of foods, supplying essential nutrients like omega-3 fatty acids, high-quality protein, vitamins (such as B12 and D), and minerals (including selenium and potassium). These nutrients are vital for heart health, brain function, and overall well-being, making this dish not only flavorful but also highly beneficial for your health.

Ingredients:
To prepare Baked Salmon with Lemon and Dill, you will need:
i. Salmon fillets: 4 (about 6 ounces each)

ii. Lemon: 1, thinly sliced
iii. Fresh dill: 2 tablespoons, chopped
iv. Olive oil: 2 tablespoons
v. Garlic: 2 cloves, minced
vi. Salt and pepper: to taste
vii. Lemon juice: 1 tablespoon, freshly squeezed

Cooking Methods:
- **Preheat the Oven:** Start by preheating your oven to 375°F (190°C). This will ensure that the oven is hot enough to cook the salmon evenly and thoroughly.
- **Prepare the Baking Dish:** Lightly grease a baking dish with a little olive oil to prevent the salmon from sticking. You can also line the dish with parchment paper for easier cleanup.
- **Season the Salmon:** Place the salmon fillets in the baking dish, skin-side down if the skin is still on. Drizzle the fillets with olive oil and freshly squeezed lemon juice. Sprinkle minced garlic, salt, and pepper evenly over the salmon.
- **Add Lemon and Dill:** Lay thin slices of lemon over each salmon fillet. Sprinkle chopped fresh dill generously over the top. The lemon slices will infuse the salmon with a bright citrus flavor, while the dill adds a fragrant, herbaceous note.
- **Bake the Salmon:** Place the baking dish in the preheated oven. Bake the salmon for 15-20 minutes, or until the salmon flakes easily with a fork. The exact cooking time will depend on the

thickness of the fillets, but the general rule is to bake for about 10 minutes per inch of thickness.

- **Serve:** Once the salmon is done, remove it from the oven and let it rest for a couple of minutes. This allows the juices to redistribute, keeping the salmon moist and flavorful. Serve the baked salmon fillets hot, garnished with additional fresh dill and lemon wedges if desired.

Baked Salmon with Lemon and Dill is a quick and straightforward dish, taking about 20-25 minutes from start to finish, including preparation and cooking time. This recipe serves four, making it an excellent choice for a family dinner or a gathering with friends. Each serving provides a substantial amount of protein, heart-healthy fats, and essential vitamins and minerals, contributing to a balanced and nutritious meal. Enjoy this dish with a side of steamed vegetables, quinoa, or a fresh salad to complete your healthy and satisfying dinner.

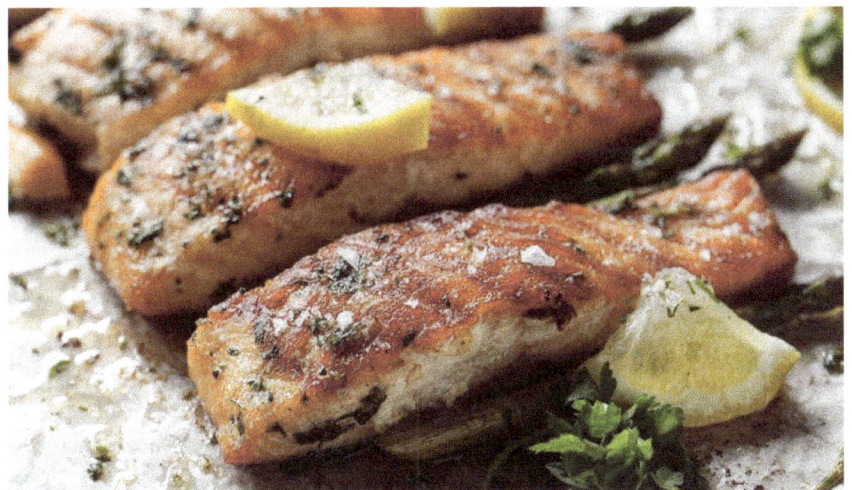
Baked Salmon With Lemon And Dill

■ Grilled Chicken With Herbed Quinoa

Grilled Chicken with Herbed Quinoa is a flavorful and nutritious dish that perfectly balances protein, grains, and fresh herbs. This meal features tender, juicy grilled chicken paired with a fragrant and wholesome herbed quinoa. Chicken, a rich source of high-quality protein, supports muscle repair and growth, while quinoa, a complete grain, provides essential amino acids, fiber, and minerals like magnesium and iron. Fresh herbs not only enhance the dish's flavor but also add antioxidants and vitamins, making this a well-rounded, nutrient-dense option for those looking to maintain a healthy, Candida-friendly diet.

Ingredients:

For the Grilled Chicken:
i. Chicken breasts: 4, boneless and skinless
ii. Olive oil: 2 tablespoons
iii. Lemon juice: 2 tablespoons
iv. Garlic: 2 cloves, minced
v. Fresh rosemary: 1 tablespoon, chopped
vi. Fresh thyme: 1 tablespoon, chopped
vii. Salt and pepper: to taste

For the Herbed Quinoa:
viii. Quinoa: 1 cup, rinsed
ix. Water or chicken broth: 2 cups
x. Olive oil: 1 tablespoon
xi. Fresh parsley: 1/4 cup, chopped
xii. Fresh cilantro: 1/4 cup, chopped
xiii. Lemon zest: 1 teaspoon
xiv. Salt and pepper: to taste

Cooking Methods:
- **Marinate the Chicken:** In a bowl, combine the olive oil, lemon juice, minced garlic, chopped rosemary, thyme, salt, and pepper. Add the chicken breasts, ensuring they are well-coated with the marinade. Cover and let marinate in the refrigerator for at least 30 minutes, or up to 2 hours for deeper flavor.
- **Cook the Quinoa:** In a medium saucepan, bring the water or chicken broth to a boil. Add the rinsed quinoa, reduce the heat to low, cover, and simmer for about 15 minutes, or until the quinoa is tender and the liquid is absorbed. Remove from

heat and let it sit, covered, for 5 minutes. Fluff with a fork.
- **Prepare the Herbed Quinoa:** In a large bowl, mix the cooked quinoa with olive oil, chopped parsley, cilantro, lemon zest, salt, and pepper. Toss well to combine all the flavors.
- **Grill the Chicken:** Preheat the grill to medium-high heat. Remove the chicken from the marinade and grill for about 6-7 minutes on each side, or until the internal temperature reaches 165°F (75°C) and the chicken is cooked through with clear juices. Let the chicken rest for a few minutes before slicing.

Grilled Chicken with Herbed Quinoa takes approximately 45 minutes to prepare, including marinating and cooking time. This recipe serves four people, making it an ideal choice for a family dinner or a small gathering. The grilled chicken offers a juicy, flavorful protein source, while the herbed quinoa provides a light, fragrant accompaniment rich in fiber and essential nutrients. Together, they create a balanced, satisfying meal that supports overall health and well-being. Enjoy this delightful dish as part of your Candida-friendly lifestyle, knowing you are nourishing your body with wholesome, delicious food.

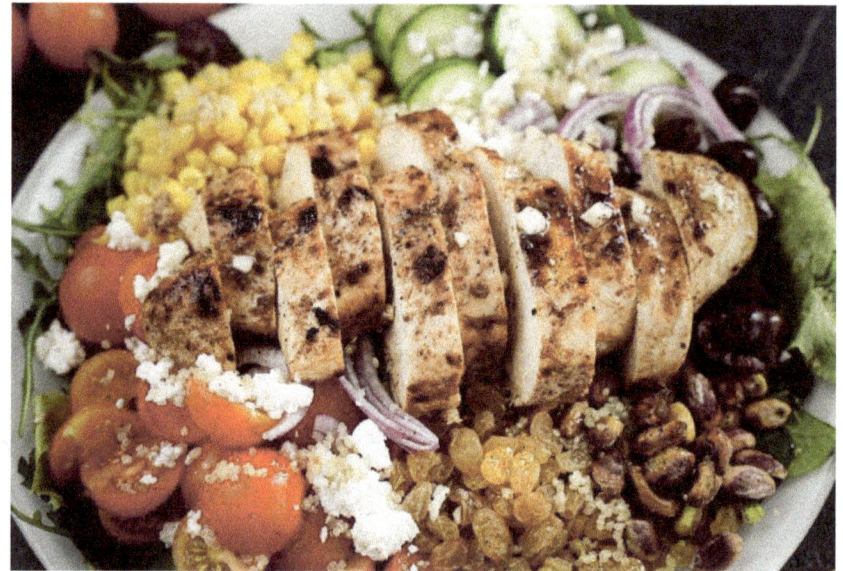
Grilled Chickens With Herbed Quinoa

■ Lentil And Vegetable Stir-Fry

Lentil and Vegetable Stir-Fry combines the protein-rich goodness of lentils with a variety of fresh vegetables. This stir-fry not only bursts with flavor but also provides a well-rounded meal, featuring proteins, carbohydrates, fiber, and essential vitamins and minerals. Lentils, a member of the legume family, are an excellent source of plant-based protein and fiber, while the colorful vegetables supply a range of vitamins, minerals, and antioxidants. This dish is perfect for those seeking a wholesome, balanced meal that supports a Candida-friendly diet.

Ingredients:

For the Lentil and Vegetable Stir-Fry, you will need:

i. Lentils: 1 cup, cooked
ii. Olive oil: 2 tablespoons
iii. Onion: 1 medium, chopped
iv. Garlic: 3 cloves, minced
v. Carrots: 2, sliced
vi. Bell peppers: 2 (any color), sliced
vii. Broccoli florets: 2 cups
viii. Zucchini: 1, sliced
ix. Soy sauce or tamari: 3 tablespoons
x. Fresh ginger: 1 tablespoon, grated
xi. Lemon juice: 2 tablespoons
xii. Fresh cilantro: 1/4 cup, chopped (optional for garnish)
xiii. Salt and pepper: to taste

Cooking Methods:

- **Prepare the Lentils:** Rinse the lentils under cold water. In a pot, combine lentils with water and bring to a boil. Reduce the heat and simmer for about 20-25 minutes, or until tender. Drain any excess water and set the lentils aside.
- **Sauté Aromatics:** In a large skillet or wok, heat olive oil over medium heat. Add the chopped onion and minced garlic, sautéing until fragrant and translucent, about 3-4 minutes.
- **Add Vegetables:** Add the sliced carrots, bell peppers, broccoli florets, and zucchini to the skillet. Stir-fry the vegetables for about 5-7 minutes, or until they are tender-crisp.

- ➢ **Combine Lentils and Seasonings:** Add the cooked lentils to the skillet, mixing them with the vegetables. Pour in the soy sauce or tamari, grated fresh ginger, and lemon juice. Stir well to combine and cook for an additional 2-3 minutes, allowing the flavors to meld together.
- ➢ **Season and Garnish:** Season the stir-fry with salt and pepper to taste. If desired, garnish with freshly chopped cilantro for a burst of fresh flavor.

The Lentil and Vegetable Stir-Fry can be prepared in about 30-35 minutes, including the time to cook the lentils. This recipe serves approximately four people, making it a great option for a family meal or meal prep for the week. Each serving provides a hearty portion of protein, fiber, and a variety of essential nutrients, ensuring a balanced and satisfying meal. Enjoy this stir-fry on its own or over a bed of quinoa or brown rice for an extra boost of whole grains. This dish is not only delicious but also supports your journey towards better health and well-being on a Candida-friendly diet.

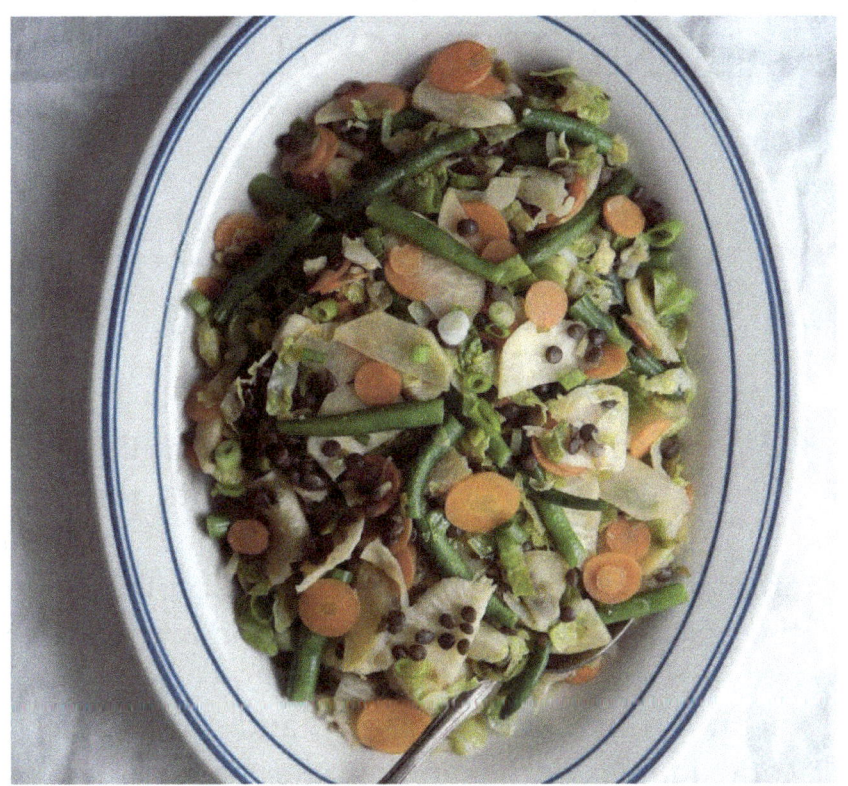

Lentil And Vegetable Stir-Fry

COMFORTING VEGETABLE DISHES

■ Roasted Garlic Brussels Sprouts

Roasted Garlic Brussels Sprout is a nutritious side dish that brings out the natural sweetness of Brussels sprouts through the roasting process, complemented by the rich, aromatic flavor of garlic. Brussels sprouts belong to the cruciferous vegetable family and are packed with essential nutrients. They provide a good source of dietary fiber, vitamins C and K, folate, and antioxidants. Garlic, on the other hand, is known for its immune-boosting properties and adds a depth of flavor to the dish. This combination not only makes for a tasty treat but also supports overall health and well-being, making it a perfect addition to a balanced diet.

Ingredients:

To make Roasted Garlic Brussels Sprouts, you will need:
i. Brussels sprouts: 1 pound, trimmed and halved
ii. Garlic cloves: 4-5, minced
iii. Olive oil: 2-3 tablespoons
iv. Salt: to taste
v. Black pepper: to taste

vi. Lemon juice: 1 tablespoon (optional, for added brightness)
vii. Parmesan cheese: 1/4 cup, grated (optional, for garnish)

Cooking Methods:
- **Preheat the Oven:** Start by preheating your oven to 400°F (200°C). This ensures that the Brussels sprouts will roast evenly and develop a nice, crispy exterior.
- **Prepare the Brussels Sprouts:** Trim the ends of the Brussels sprouts and remove any yellow or damaged outer leaves. Cut each sprout in half to ensure they cook evenly. Place the halved Brussels sprouts in a large mixing bowl
- **Add Garlic and Seasonings:** Mince the garlic cloves and add them to the bowl with the Brussels sprouts. Drizzle the olive oil over the sprouts, ensuring they are evenly coated. Season with salt and black pepper to taste. Toss everything together until the Brussels sprouts are well coated with the garlic, oil, and seasonings.
- **Roast the Brussels Sprouts:** Spread the seasoned Brussels sprouts in a single layer on a baking sheet. This helps them roast evenly and get crispy. Place the baking sheet in the preheated oven and roast for 20-25 minutes, stirring halfway through. The Brussels sprouts should be tender on the inside and caramelized on the outside.
- **Finish and Serve:** Once roasted, remove the Brussels sprouts from the oven and transfer them

to a serving bowl. If desired, drizzle with fresh lemon juice for a touch of brightness. For an extra layer of flavor, sprinkle grated Parmesan cheese over the top.

Roasted Garlic Brussels Sprouts are ready in about 30-35 minutes, including prep and cooking time. This recipe serves about four people as a side dish. The roasting process enhances the natural flavors of the Brussels sprouts, making them sweet and caramelized, while the garlic adds a savory note. The optional lemon juice and Parmesan cheese elevate the dish, adding a burst of freshness and a hint of umami. Enjoy these Roasted Garlic Brussels Sprouts alongside your favorite protein or as a delicious addition to any meal, providing a wholesome, flavorful, and nutrient-dense option for your diet.

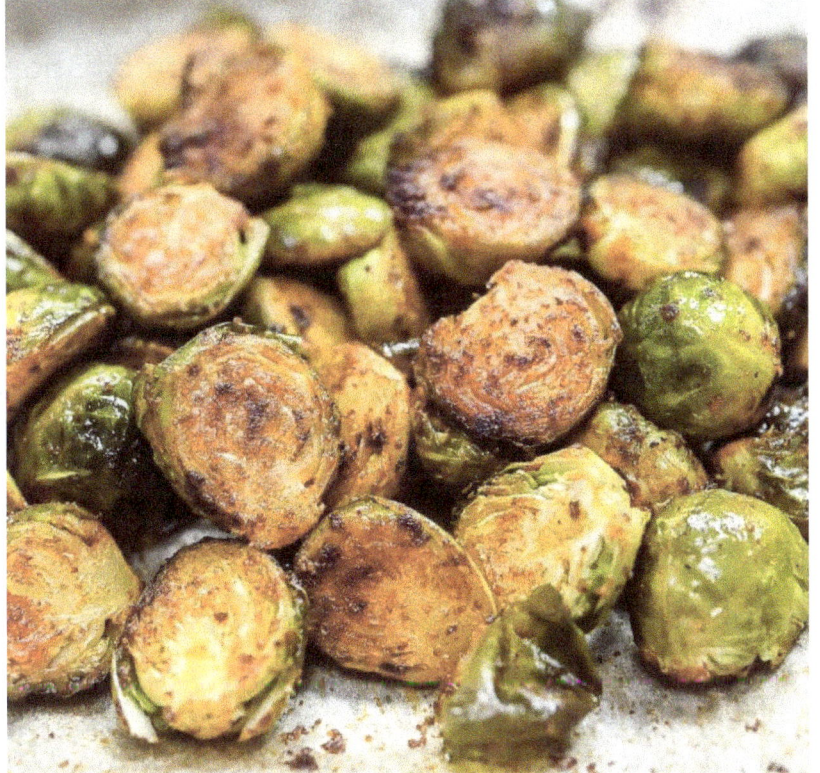

Roasted Garlic Brussels Sprouts

■ Zucchini Noodles With Pesto

Zucchini Noodles with Pesto readily brings together the freshness of zucchini with the rich, aromatic flavors of homemade pesto. This dish is a fantastic low-carb alternative to traditional pasta, making it perfect for those looking to manage Candida overgrowth or simply reduce their intake of refined carbohydrates. Zucchini noodles provide essential vitamins and minerals, while the pesto, made from fresh basil, nuts, and olive oil, offers healthy fats and antioxidants. This combination not only creates a tasty meal but also supports overall health and well-being.

Ingredients:

For the Zucchini Noodles:
i. Zucchini: 4 medium-sized, spiralized into noodles
ii. Olive oil: 1 tablespoon
iii. Salt: to taste

For the Pesto:
iv. Fresh basil leaves: 2 cups, packed
v. Pine nuts or walnuts: 1/4 cup
vi. Garlic: 2 cloves
vii. Parmesan cheese: 1/4 cup, grated (optional)
viii. Lemon juice: 1 tablespoon
ix. Olive oil: 1/3 cup
x. Salt and pepper: to taste

Cooking Methods:

- **Prepare the Zucchini Noodles:** Start by washing the zucchini thoroughly. Using a spiralizer, create long noodles from the zucchini. If you don't have a spiralizer, you can use a vegetable peeler to make thin ribbons or julienne the zucchini into thin strips.
- **Make the Pesto:** In a food processor, combine the fresh basil leaves, pine nuts or walnuts, garlic cloves, and grated Parmesan cheese (if using).

Pulse until the ingredients are finely chopped. Add the lemon juice and continue to pulse while slowly drizzling in the olive oil until the mixture reaches a smooth, creamy consistency. Season with salt and pepper to taste.
- **Cook the Zucchini Noodles:** In a large skillet, heat the olive oil over medium heat. Add the zucchini noodles and sauté for 2-3 minutes, just until they are tender but still slightly firm (al dente). Season with a pinch of salt.
- **Combine and Serve:** Remove the skillet from heat and add the pesto to the zucchini noodles. Toss gently to ensure the noodles are evenly coated with the pesto.

This Zucchini Noodles with Pesto dish comes together quickly, with a total preparation and cooking time of about 15-20 minutes. It serves approximately four people, making it an excellent choice for a quick weeknight dinner or a light, nutritious lunch. Each serving is a powerhouse of nutrients: the zucchini provides vitamins A and C, potassium, and fiber, while the pesto offers healthy fats from the olive oil and nuts, along with the antioxidant benefits of fresh basil. Enjoy this flavorful and wholesome dish as a satisfying meal that supports your health and dietary goals.

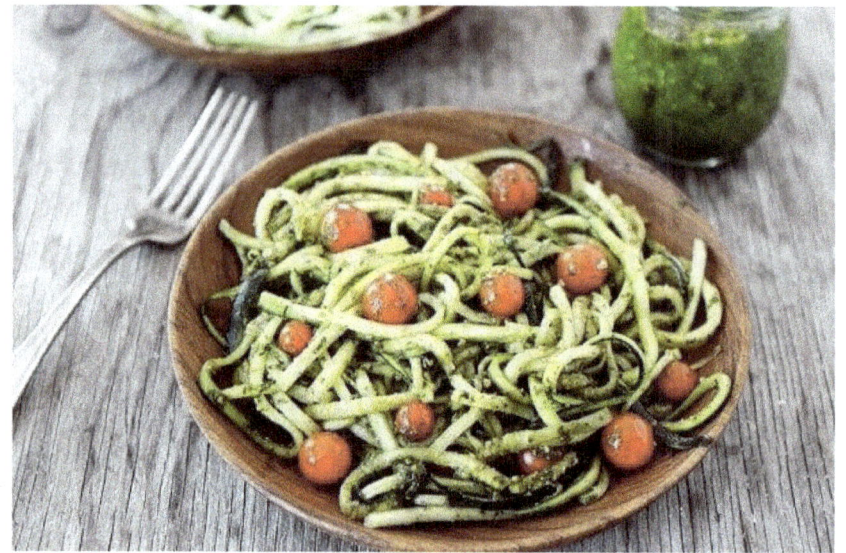
Zucchini Noodles With Pesto

■ Stuffed Bell Peppers With Brown Rice And Beans

Stuffed Bell Peppers with Brown Rice and Beans combines a variety of food classes, including vegetables, grains, and legumes. This dish is a great source of essential nutrients: bell peppers provide vitamins A and C along with antioxidants, brown rice offers complex carbohydrates and fiber, and beans contribute protein and additional fiber. Together, these ingredients create a well-balanced meal that supports overall health and fits well into a Candida-friendly diet by emphasizing whole, nutrient-dense foods.

Ingredients:

For the Stuffed Bell Peppers, you will need:
i. Bell peppers: 4 large, any color
ii. Brown rice: 1 cup, cooked
iii. Black beans: 1 cup, cooked and drained
iv. Onion: 1 medium, chopped
v. Garlic: 2 cloves, minced
vi. Tomato sauce: 1 cup
vii. Olive oil: 2 tablespoons
viii. Ground cumin: 1 teaspoon
ix. Chili powder: 1 teaspoon
x. Salt and pepper: to taste
xi. Fresh cilantro or parsley: 1/4 cup, chopped (optional for garnish)
xii. Shredded cheese: 1/2 cup (optional for topping)

Cooking Methods:

- **Prepare the Peppers:** Preheat your oven to 375°F (190°C). Cut the tops off the bell peppers and remove the seeds and membranes. If needed, trim the bottoms slightly so they stand upright. Place the peppers in a baking dish.
- **Cook the Filling:** In a large skillet, heat the olive oil over medium heat. Add the chopped onion and minced garlic, sautéing until they become translucent and fragrant, about 3-4 minutes. Stir in the cooked brown rice and black beans, mixing well to combine.
- **Season and Combine:** Add the tomato sauce, ground cumin, chili powder, salt, and pepper to the rice and bean mixture. Stir well to ensure everything is evenly coated with the spices and

- ➤ sauce. Cook for an additional 5 minutes, allowing the flavors to meld together.
- ➤ **Stuff the Peppers:** Spoon the rice and bean mixture into the prepared bell peppers, packing it down slightly to fill each pepper completely. If desired, top each stuffed pepper with a sprinkle of shredded cheese.
- ➤ **Bake:** Cover the baking dish with aluminum foil and bake in the preheated oven for 30 minutes. After 30 minutes, remove the foil and bake for an additional 10-15 minutes, until the peppers are tender and the cheese (if used) is melted and bubbly.
- ➤ **Garnish and Serve:** Once done, remove the stuffed peppers from the oven and let them cool slightly before serving. Garnish with chopped fresh cilantro or parsley if desired.

This Stuffed Bell Peppers with Brown Rice and Beans recipe requires about 15 minutes of preparation time and 45 minutes of cooking time, making it a manageable dish that can be ready in just about an hour. This recipe makes four servings, with each stuffed pepper providing a balanced combination of protein, fiber, vitamins, and minerals. Perfect as a satisfying main course, these stuffed peppers are a delicious way to enjoy a nutrient-rich meal that supports a healthy diet and fits well into a Candida-friendly eating plan. Enjoy these stuffed peppers fresh from the oven, savoring the blend of flavors and textures in every bite.

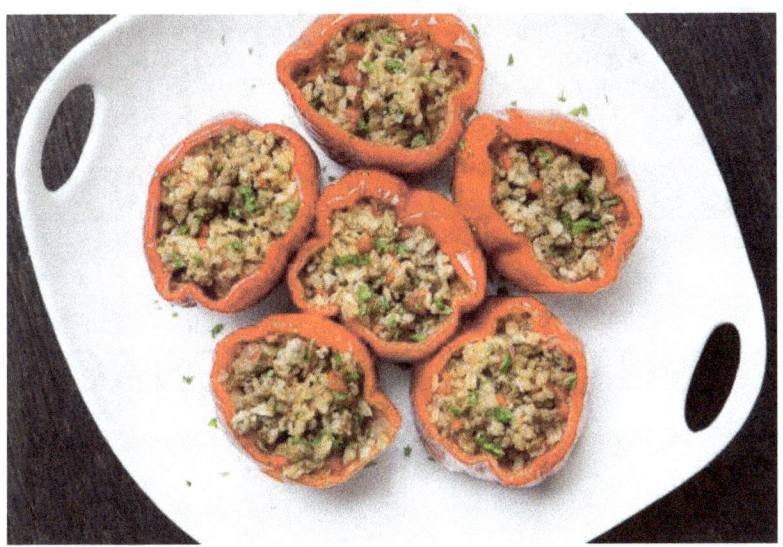

Stuffed Bell Peppers With Brown Rice And Beans

CHAPTER FOUR
TASTY SNACKS AND DISHES

NUTRIENT-RICH SNACK IDEAS

■ Almond Butter And Apple Slices

Almond Butter and Apple Slices is a simple snack that perfectly balances taste and health benefits. This delightful combination brings together the rich, creamy texture of almond butter with the crisp, refreshing crunch of apple slices. Not only is this snack quick and easy to prepare, but it also offers a powerhouse of nutrients. Almond butter provides healthy fats, protein, and fiber, while apples are a great source of vitamins, particularly vitamin C, and dietary fiber. This snack fits well into various classes of food, providing a balanced mix of macronutrients and essential vitamins and minerals.

Ingredients:

For this nutritious snack, you will need:
i. Almond butter: 2 tablespoons
ii. Apples: 1 or 2 medium-sized, preferably organic

Cooking Methods:
Prepare the Apples: Wash the apples thoroughly under running water. Using a sharp knife or an apple slicer, core the apples and slice them into even wedges. Depending on the size of the apple, you should get about 8-12 slices per apple.
Serve with Almond Butter: Place the apple slices on a serving plate. In a small bowl or directly on the plate, serve the almond butter for dipping. You can spread the almond butter directly onto the apple slices or dip them as you eat.

This snack is incredibly quick to prepare, taking only about 5 minutes from start to finish. It's a convenient option for busy days or when you need a quick, nutritious bite. Each serving, which consists of one apple paired with about two tablespoons of almond butter, makes for a satisfying snack that can be enjoyed at any time of the day. This combination provides a balanced mix of carbohydrates from the apples and healthy fats and protein from the almond butter, making it an excellent choice for maintaining steady energy levels and curbing hunger between meals. Enjoy this wholesome snack as a part of your Candida-friendly diet to keep your body nourished and energized!

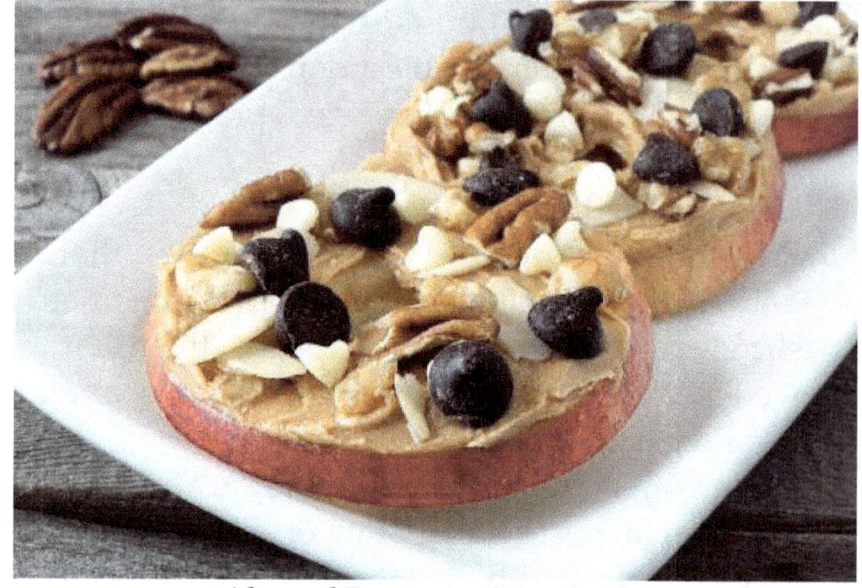

Almond Butter And Apple Slices

■ Roasted Chickpeas With Spices

Roasted Chickpeas with Spices are a delightful snack that can easily become a staple in your Candida-friendly diet. Chickpeas, also known as garbanzo beans, are a member of the legume family and are packed with essential nutrients. They are an excellent source of protein, making them a great plant-based protein option, especially for vegetarians and vegans. Chickpeas also provide a good amount of dietary fiber, which supports digestive health and helps maintain stable blood sugar levels. Additionally, they contain important vitamins and minerals, including iron, magnesium, and folate. When roasted with a blend of flavorful spices, chickpeas transform into a crunchy, savory snack that's both satisfying and healthy.

Ingredients:

To make Roasted Chickpeas with Spices, you will need:

i. Canned chickpeas: 1 can (15 ounces), drained and rinsed
ii. Olive oil: 2 tablespoons
iii. Ground cumin: 1 teaspoon
iv. Ground paprika: 1 teaspoon
v. Garlic powder: 1/2 teaspoon
vi. Salt: 1/2 teaspoon
vii. Ground black pepper: 1/4 teaspoon
viii. Optional: cayenne pepper or chili powder for a spicy kick, 1/4 teaspoon

Cooking Methods:

- **Preheat the Oven:** Preheat your oven to 400°F (200°C).
- **Prepare the Chickpeas:** After draining and rinsing the canned chickpeas, spread them out on a clean kitchen towel or paper towels. Pat them dry thoroughly. Removing as much moisture as possible will help them roast evenly and become crispier.
- **Season the Chickpeas:** Transfer the dried chickpeas to a large mixing bowl. Add the olive oil, ground cumin, ground paprika, garlic powder, salt, and ground black pepper. If you prefer a spicier flavor, add cayenne pepper or chili

powder. Toss the chickpeas well to ensure they are evenly coated with the oil and spices.
- **Roast the Chickpeas:** Spread the seasoned chickpeas in a single layer on a baking sheet. Make sure they are not too crowded, as this will help them roast more evenly. Place the baking sheet in the preheated oven.
- **Bake and Stir:** Roast the chickpeas for about 25-30 minutes, stirring them once or twice during cooking to ensure they roast evenly. Keep an eye on them towards the end to prevent burning. They should be golden brown and crispy when done.
- **Cool and Serve:** Once roasted, remove the chickpeas from the oven and let them cool on the baking sheet for a few minutes. They will continue to crisp up as they cool. Serve them warm or at room temperature as a snack, or sprinkle them over salads for added crunch and flavor.

The total cooking time for Roasted Chickpeas with Spices is approximately 30-35 minutes, including preparation and roasting. This recipe makes about 4 servings, making it an ideal snack for a small group or a batch to enjoy over a few days. Roasted chickpeas can be stored in an airtight container at room temperature for up to a week, although they are best enjoyed fresh for maximum crunchiness. This simple yet flavorful snack is a fantastic way to enjoy the health benefits of chickpeas while sticking to a Candida-friendly diet.

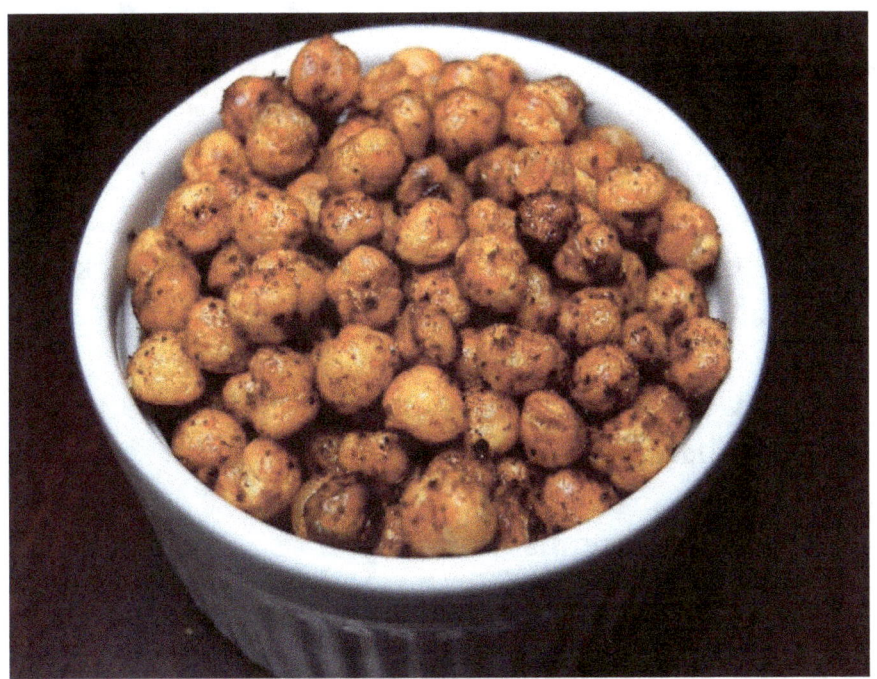

Roasted Chicken peas with spicies

■ Raw Veggie Sticks With Hummus

Raw Veggie Sticks with Hummus is a simple snack that brings together the crisp freshness of raw vegetables with the creamy richness of hummus. This dish is a great way to incorporate various classes of food into your diet. The vegetables provide essential vitamins, minerals, and fiber, while hummus, made from chickpeas, tahini, olive oil, and lemon juice, offers a good source of protein, healthy fats, and additional vitamins. This combination makes for a balanced and satisfying snack, perfect for anyone looking to maintain a healthy and Candida-friendly diet.

Ingredients:

For the Raw Veggie Sticks:
i. Carrots: 2 large, peeled and cut into sticks
ii. Celery: 2 stalks, washed and cut into sticks
iii. Bell peppers: 2 (one red, one yellow), seeded and sliced into sticks
iv. Cucumber: 1 medium, peeled and cut into sticks
v. Cherry tomatoes: 1 cup, washed

For the Hummus:
vi. Chickpeas: 1 can (15 oz), drained and rinsed
vii. Tahini: 1/4 cup
viii. Olive oil: 2 tablespoons
ix. Lemon juice: 2 tablespoons, freshly squeezed
x. Garlic: 1 clove, minced
xi. Salt: 1/2 teaspoon
xii. Water: 2-3 tablespoons (as needed for desired consistency)

Cooking Methods:
➢ **Prepare the Veggie Sticks:** Begin by washing and preparing all the vegetables. Peel and cut the carrots and cucumber into sticks. Wash and cut the celery stalks into sticks. Seed and slice the bell peppers into strips. Rinse the cherry tomatoes and

pat them dry. Arrange all the prepared vegetables on a serving platter.
- **Make the Hummus:** In a food processor, combine the drained chickpeas, tahini, olive oil, lemon juice, minced garlic, and salt. Blend until smooth. If the hummus is too thick, add water, one tablespoon at a time, until you reach the desired consistency. Taste and adjust the seasoning as needed.
- **Serve:** Transfer the hummus to a small serving bowl and place it in the center of the platter with the veggie sticks. You can drizzle a little olive oil on top of the hummus and sprinkle some paprika or chopped fresh parsley for garnish, if desired.

The preparation for Raw Veggie Sticks with Hummus is quick and straightforward, taking approximately 20 minutes to complete. This recipe serves about four people, making it an excellent choice for a healthy snack, appetizer, or a light lunch. The variety of fresh vegetables paired with the creamy, flavorful hummus provides a delightful contrast in textures and flavors, ensuring that this dish is both satisfying and nutritious. Enjoy this vibrant and healthy snack as part of your Candida-friendly diet and relish the benefits of wholesome, natural foods.

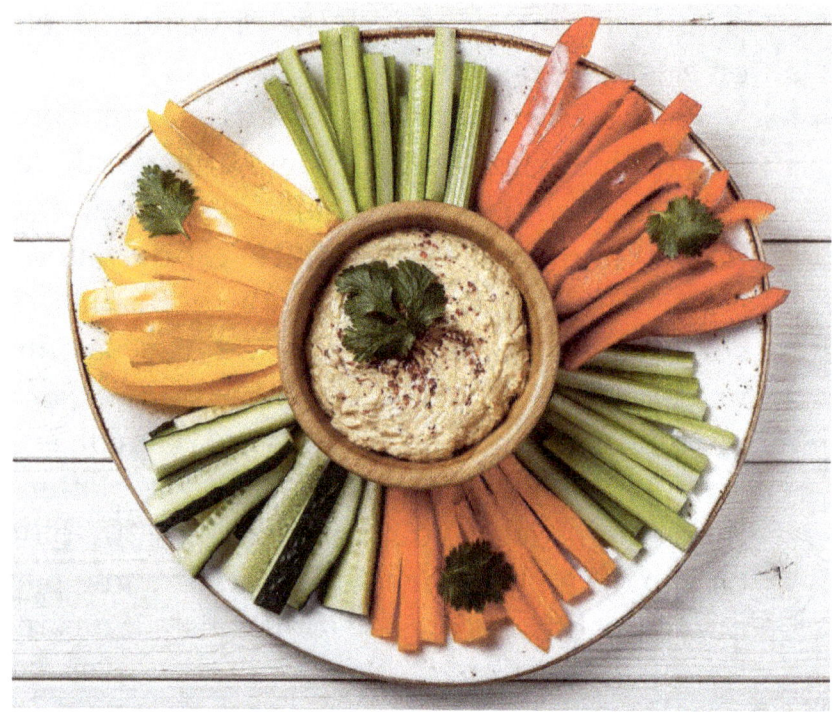

Raw Veggie Sticks With Hummus

CANDIDA OVERGROWTH TREATMENT

FLAVORFUL SIDE DISHES

■ Garlic And Herb Quinoa

Garlic and Herb Quinoa serves as an excellent side course. Quinoa, a superfood, is a gluten-free grain that belongs to the seed class of foods. It is packed with protein, fiber, vitamins, and minerals. This dish combines the nutty flavor of quinoa with the aromatic blend of garlic and fresh herbs, providing a satisfying and healthy option for any meal. Quinoa is a complete protein, meaning it contains all nine essential amino acids, making it a valuable addition to a balanced diet. It also supplies magnesium, iron, and B vitamins, contributing to overall health and well-being.

Ingredients:

For Garlic and Herb Quinoa, you will need:
i. Quinoa: 1 cup, rinsed
ii. Vegetable broth or water: 2 cups
iii. Olive oil: 2 tablespoons
iv. Garlic cloves: 3, minced
v. Fresh parsley: 1/4 cup, chopped
vi. Fresh basil: 1/4 cup, chopped
vii. Fresh thyme: 1 tablespoon, chopped
viii. Lemon juice: 2 tablespoons
ix. Salt and pepper: to taste

Cooking Methods:

- ➤ **Prepare the Quinoa:** Begin by rinsing the quinoa under cold water to remove its natural saponin coating, which can make it taste bitter. This step ensures a clean, mild flavor.
- ➤ **Cook the Quinoa:** In a medium saucepan, bring the vegetable broth or water to a boil. Add the rinsed quinoa, reduce the heat to low, and cover. Let it simmer for about 15 minutes, or until all the liquid is absorbed and the quinoa is tender. Remove from heat and let it sit, covered, for an additional 5 minutes. Fluff with a fork to separate the grains.
- ➤ **Sauté the Garlic:** While the quinoa is cooking, heat the olive oil in a small pan over medium heat. Add the minced garlic and sauté until it becomes fragrant and lightly golden, about 1-2 minutes. Be careful not to burn the garlic, as this can impart a bitter taste.
- ➤ **Combine Ingredients:** In a large bowl, combine the cooked quinoa, sautéed garlic, chopped parsley, basil, and thyme. Drizzle with lemon juice and season with salt and pepper to taste. Toss everything together until well mixed and evenly coated with the herbs and lemon juice.

Garlic and Herb Quinoa takes about 25-30 minutes to prepare, making it a quick and easy addition to any meal. This recipe yields approximately four servings, perfect for a family dinner or meal prep for the week. Each serving is a nutrient-dense powerhouse, providing a healthy dose of protein, fiber, and essential vitamins and minerals. Enjoy this dish as a side to grilled vegetables, lean proteins, or as a standalone vegetarian meal. Its fresh, herbaceous flavors and satisfying texture make it a versatile and delightful choice for those seeking nutritious and delicious options.

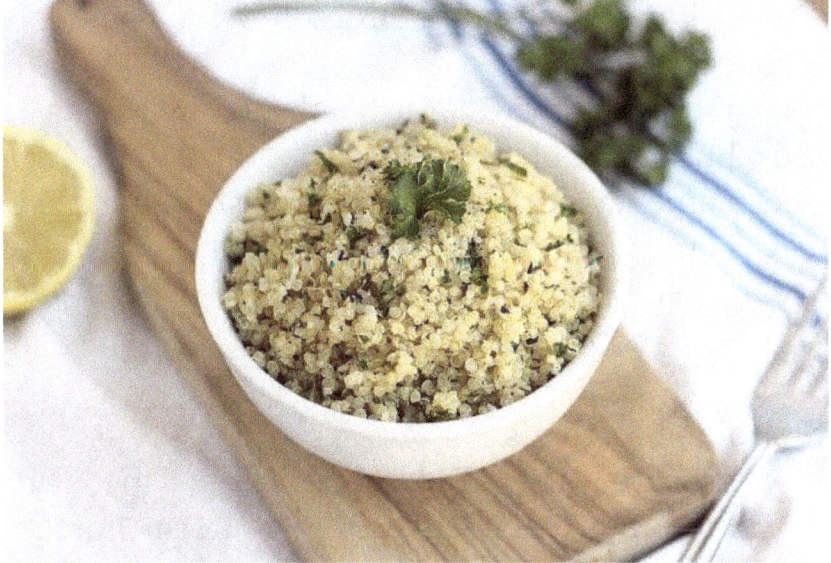

Garlic And Herb Quinoa

▪ Steamed Broccoli With Lemon Butter Sauce

Steamed Broccoli with Lemon Butter Sauce brings out the best in this nutritious vegetable. Broccoli is a member of the cruciferous vegetable family, which also includes kale, cauliflower, and Brussels sprouts. It is renowned for its high nutrient content, providing a wealth of vitamins (such as vitamin C and vitamin K), minerals (like potassium and calcium), fiber, and antioxidants. This dish combines the health benefits of broccoli with the rich, tangy flavor of a lemon butter sauce, making it both a delicious and nutritious addition to your Candida-friendly diet.

Ingredients:

For the Steamed Broccoli with Lemon Butter Sauce, you will need:

i. Fresh broccoli: 1 large head, cut into florets
ii. Butter: 3 tablespoons
iii. Lemon juice: 2 tablespoons, freshly squeezed
iv. Lemon zest: 1 teaspoon
v. Garlic: 2 cloves, minced
vi. Salt and pepper: to taste

Cooking Methods:

- **Prepare the Broccoli:** Wash the broccoli thoroughly and cut it into uniform florets. This ensures even cooking and helps maintain a pleasant texture.
- **Steam the Broccoli:** In a large pot with a steamer basket, bring a few inches of water to a boil. Place the broccoli florets in the steamer basket, cover, and steam for about 5-7 minutes, or until the broccoli is tender but still vibrant green. Be careful not to overcook the broccoli, as it should retain some crunch.

- ➢ **Make the Lemon Butter Sauce:** While the broccoli is steaming, prepare the lemon butter sauce. In a small saucepan over medium heat, melt the butter. Add the minced garlic and sauté for about 1-2 minutes, until fragrant. Remove from heat and stir in the freshly squeezed lemon juice and lemon zest. Season with salt and pepper to taste.
- ➢ **Combine and Serve:** Once the broccoli is done steaming, transfer it to a serving bowl. Drizzle the lemon butter sauce over the steamed broccoli, tossing gently to ensure even coating. Adjust the seasoning if necessary.

The entire process of making Steamed Broccoli with Lemon Butter Sauce takes about 15-20 minutes, making it a quick and easy side dish option. This recipe serves approximately four people, making it perfect for a family dinner or as a healthy addition to any meal. The bright, fresh flavors of the lemon butter sauce perfectly complement the natural sweetness of the broccoli, creating a dish that is both satisfying and packed with nutrients. Enjoy this dish as a part of your balanced, Candida-friendly diet, knowing that you are fueling your body with wholesome, delicious food.

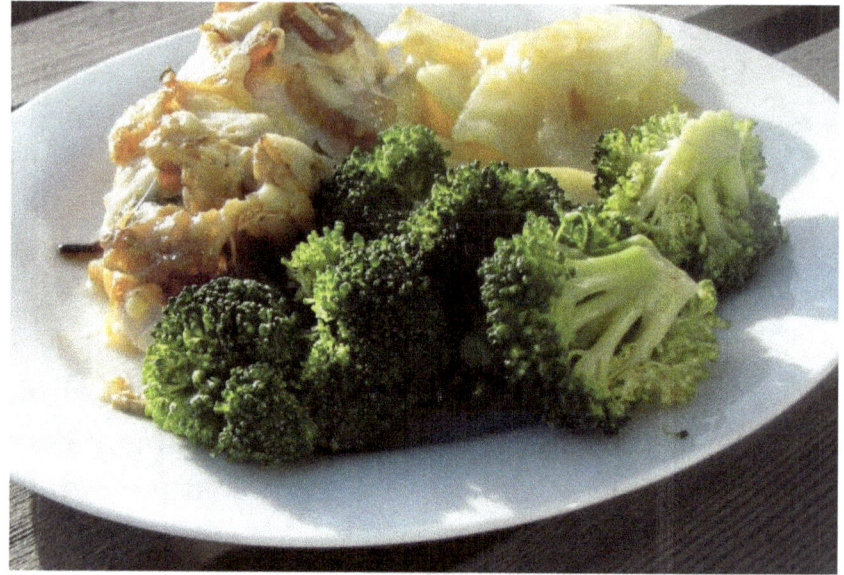

Steamed Broccoli With Lemon Butter Sauce

■ Mashed Cauliflower With Roasted Garlic

Mashed Cauliflower with Roasted Garlic is a an alternative to traditional mashed potatoes. This dish combines the creamy texture of cauliflower with the rich, savory flavor of roasted garlic, making it a perfect side dish for any meal. Cauliflower belongs to the cruciferous vegetable family and is packed with essential nutrients, including vitamins C, K, and B6, folate, and fiber. This dish also provides healthy fats from the olive oil used in roasting the garlic, contributing to a well-rounded, nutrient-dense addition to your Candida-friendly diet.

Ingredients:

For the Mashed Cauliflower with Roasted Garlic, you will need:
i. Cauliflower: 1 large head, cut into florets
ii. Garlic: 1 whole head
iii. Olive oil: 2 tablespoons
iv. Butter or ghee: 2 tablespoons (optional, for extra creaminess)
v. Salt: to taste
vi. Black pepper: to taste
vii. Fresh parsley: 2 tablespoons, chopped (optional, for garnish)

Cooking Methods:
- **Prepare and Roast the Garlic:** Preheat your oven to 400°F (200°C). Slice the top off the head of garlic to expose the cloves. Drizzle with 1 tablespoon of olive oil and wrap it in aluminum foil. Roast in the oven for about 30-40 minutes, until the cloves are soft and golden.
- **Cook the Cauliflower**: While the garlic is roasting, bring a large pot of water to a boil. Add the cauliflower florets and cook for about 10-12 minutes, or until the cauliflower is very tender. Drain the cauliflower well and let it sit for a few minutes to release any excess moisture.
- **Mash the Cauliflower:** Transfer the cooked cauliflower to a large mixing bowl or a food processor. Squeeze the roasted garlic cloves out of their skins and add them to the cauliflower. Add the remaining 1 tablespoon of olive oil and the butter or ghee, if using. Mash the mixture with a

potato masher or blend in the food processor until smooth and creamy. Season with salt and black pepper to taste.
- **Serve:** Transfer the mashed cauliflower to a serving bowl and garnish with chopped fresh parsley if desired. Serve hot as a delicious and nutritious side dish.

The entire process for making Mashed Cauliflower with Roasted Garlic takes about 50-60 minutes, with the garlic roasting and cauliflower cooking times overlapping to save time. This recipe yields approximately four servings, making it an ideal side dish for a family meal or a small gathering. Each serving is rich in vitamins and minerals from the cauliflower, along with the added benefits of antioxidants from the roasted garlic. This dish is not only satisfying and flavorful but also aligns perfectly with a healthy, Candida-friendly diet. Enjoy this wholesome side dish as a delightful complement to your main course.

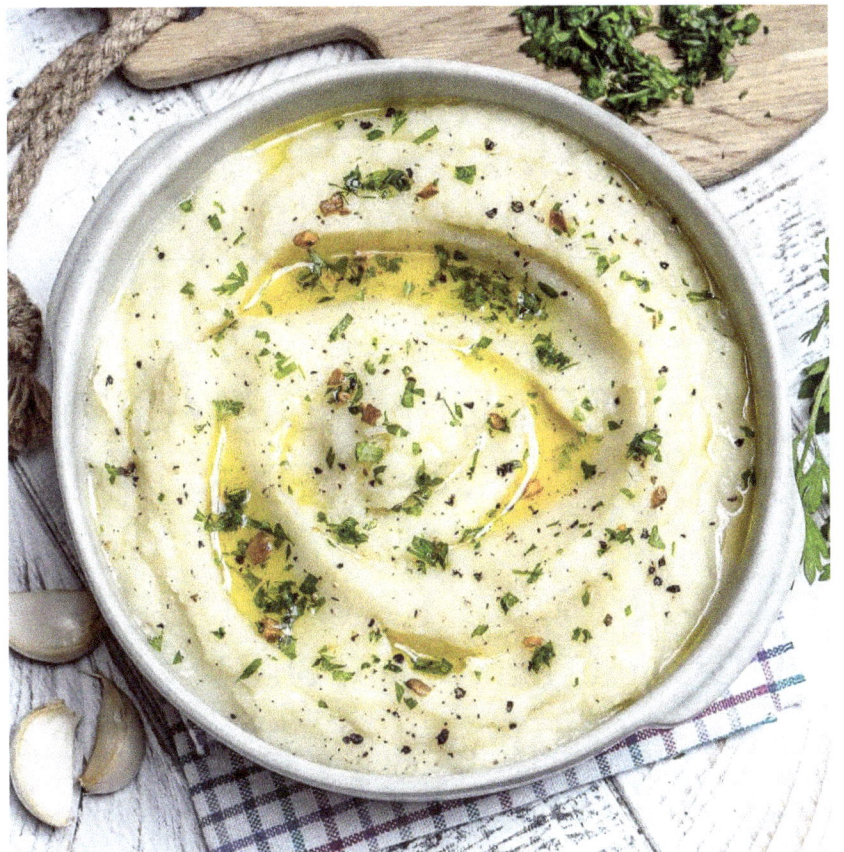

Mashed Cauliflower With Roasted Garlic

CHAPTER FIVE
SWEET TREATS AND DESSERTS

DECADENT DESSERT CREATIONS

■ Coconut Flour Banana Bread

Coconut Flour Banana Bread is a nutritious alternative to traditional banana bread, perfect for those following a Candida-friendly diet or seeking a gluten-free option. This bread combines the natural sweetness of ripe bananas with the rich, nutty flavor of coconut flour. It's packed with dietary fiber, healthy fats, and essential vitamins and minerals. This recipe is a wonderful way to enjoy a comforting treat while nourishing your body with wholesome ingredients. The bananas provide carbohydrates and potassium, the eggs contribute protein, and the coconut flour offers fiber and healthy fats, making this a balanced and satisfying food choice.

Ingredients:

For Coconut Flour Banana Bread, you will need:
i. Ripe bananas: 3 large, mashed
ii. Eggs: 4 large
iii. Coconut flour: 1/2 cup
iv. Baking soda: 1 teaspoon
v. Baking powder: 1 teaspoon
vi. Salt: 1/4 teaspoon
vii. Vanilla extract: 1 teaspoon
viii. Cinnamon: 1 teaspoon (optional for added flavor)
ix. Coconut oil: 1/4 cup, melted
x. Honey or stevia: 2 tablespoons (optional for extra sweetness)

Cooking Methods:

- **Preheat the Oven:** Preheat your oven to 350°F (175°C) and grease a loaf pan with coconut oil or line it with parchment paper for easy removal.
- **Prepare the Wet Ingredients:** In a large mixing bowl, mash the ripe bananas until smooth. Add the eggs, melted coconut oil, vanilla extract, and honey or stevia (if using). Mix well to combine all the wet ingredients.
- **Combine Dry Ingredients:** In a separate bowl, sift together the coconut flour, baking soda, baking powder, salt, and cinnamon (if using). Coconut flour can be clumpy, so sifting helps to ensure a smooth batter.
- **Mix Wet and Dry Ingredients:** Gradually add the dry ingredients to the wet mixture, stirring well

until a thick, uniform batter forms. The batter will be thicker than traditional banana bread batter due to the absorbent nature of coconut flour.
- ➤ **Pour into Loaf Pan:** Pour the batter into the prepared loaf pan, spreading it evenly with a spatula.
- ➤ **Bake:** Place the loaf pan in the preheated oven and bake for 45-55 minutes, or until a toothpick inserted into the center of the bread comes out clean. If the top starts to brown too quickly, cover it loosely with aluminum foil.
- ➤ **Cool:** Allow the banana bread to cool in the pan for about 10 minutes before transferring it to a wire rack to cool completely.

The total preparation and cooking time for Coconut Flour Banana Bread is about 1 hour. This recipe yields approximately 10 slices, making it perfect for sharing with family or enjoying throughout the week. Each slice of this banana bread is not only a delightful treat but also a nutritious one, providing a good source of dietary fiber, healthy fats, and essential vitamins and minerals. Enjoy it as a breakfast option, a snack, or even a healthy dessert. The natural sweetness of the bananas, combined with the rich texture of coconut flour, makes this bread a comforting and healthful choice for any time of the day.

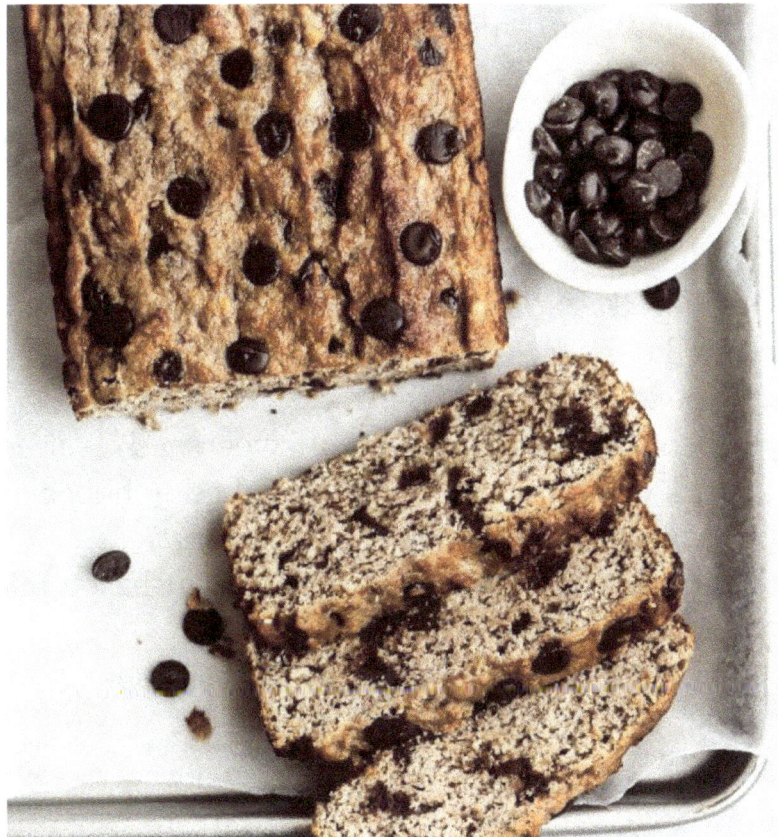
Coconut Flour Banana Bread

- ## Avocado Chocolate Mousse

Avocado Chocolate Mousse is a delectable dessert that combines the creamy texture of avocados with the rich, indulgent flavor of chocolate. This dessert not only satisfies your sweet tooth but also offers a range of nutritional benefits, making it a healthier alternative to traditional chocolate mousse. Avocados provide healthy fats, fiber, and essential vitamins, while dark chocolate contributes antioxidants and minerals. This mousse falls into the dessert category but stands out by supplying healthy fats, fiber, antioxidants, and various vitamins and minerals.

Ingredients:
For this luscious Avocado Chocolate Mousse, you will need:
i. Ripe avocados: 2 large, pitted and peeled
ii. Cocoa powder: 1/4 cup (unsweetened)
iii. Dark chocolate: 1/4 cup, melted (choose high-quality, 70% or higher cocoa content)
iv. Almond milk: 1/4 cup (or any plant-based milk of choice)
v. Honey or maple syrup: 2-4 tablespoons (adjust to taste)
vi. Vanilla extract: 1 teaspoon
vii. A pinch of salt

Cooking Methods:
- **Prepare the Avocados:** Start by scooping the flesh of the ripe avocados into a blender or food processor. Make sure the avocados are ripe and creamy to achieve the best texture for your mousse.
- **Add the Cocoa Powder and Melted Chocolate:** Add the unsweetened cocoa powder and the melted dark chocolate to the blender. The dark chocolate should be melted and slightly cooled before adding it to the mixture to ensure it blends smoothly.

- ➢ **Blend with Liquid Ingredients:** Pour in the almond milk, honey or maple syrup, and vanilla extract. Add a pinch of salt to enhance the flavors. Blend all the ingredients until smooth and creamy, stopping occasionally to scrape down the sides of the blender to ensure everything is well incorporated.
- ➢ **Adjust Sweetness and Texture:** Taste the mousse and adjust the sweetness by adding more honey or maple syrup if desired. If the mousse is too thick, add a bit more almond milk, a tablespoon at a time, until the desired consistency is achieved.
- ➢ **Chill the Mousse:** Transfer the mousse into serving bowls or glasses. Cover and refrigerate for at least 1 hour to allow the flavors to meld and the mousse to set.

The Avocado Chocolate Mousse takes about 10-15 minutes to prepare and requires at least 1 hour to chill in the refrigerator before serving. This recipe makes approximately four servings, depending on portion size. Each serving is a delightful and nutritious treat, rich in healthy fats from the avocados and antioxidants from the dark chocolate. Enjoy this mousse as a guilt-free dessert that satisfies your chocolate cravings while providing beneficial nutrients. Whether you're serving it to family, friends, or enjoying it as a personal indulgence, this Avocado Chocolate Mousse is sure to impress with its creamy texture and rich flavor.

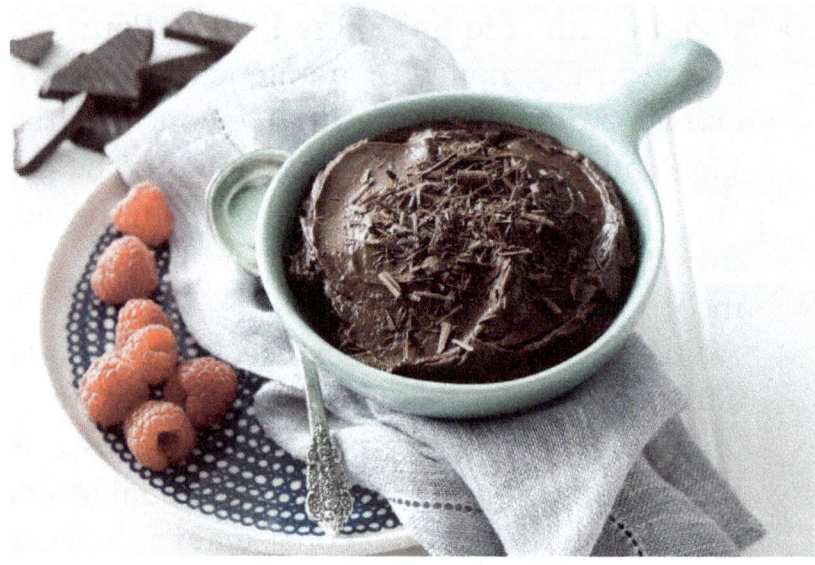
Avocado Chocolate Mousse

■ Berry Coconut Ice Pops

Berry Coconut Ice Pops are refreshing treat perfect for hot days, and they make a great addition to a Candida-friendly diet. These ice pops are not only tasty but also packed with essential nutrients. The berries provide a rich source of antioxidants, vitamins, and fiber, while the coconut milk adds healthy fats and a creamy texture. Together, they create a delightful dessert that satisfies your sweet tooth without compromising your health goals.

Ingredients:

For these nutritious ice pops, you will need:
i. Mixed berries (strawberries, blueberries, raspberries): 2 cups, fresh or frozen

ii. Coconut milk: 1 cup, full-fat for creaminess
iii. Stevia or monk fruit sweetener: 2 tablespoons, or to taste
iv. Vanilla extract: 1 teaspoon
v. Lemon juice: 1 tablespoon, freshly squeezed (optional for a tangy twist)

Cooking Methods:
Prepare the Berry Mixture: In a blender, combine the mixed berries, coconut milk, stevia or monk fruit sweetener, vanilla extract, and lemon juice (if using). Blend until smooth and well combined. If you prefer a chunkier texture, pulse the mixture a few times instead of blending it completely smooth.

Taste and Adjust: Taste the mixture and adjust the sweetness if needed by adding more stevia or monk fruit sweetener. Remember, the sweetness might mellow once frozen, so it's okay if the mixture tastes slightly sweeter than you'd like.

Pour into Molds: Pour the blended mixture into ice pop molds, leaving a small space at the top to allow for expansion as they freeze. If you don't have ice pop molds, small paper cups or an ice cube tray can work as substitutes. Insert the sticks into the molds.

Freeze: Place the filled molds in the freezer and let them freeze for at least 4-6 hours, or until completely solid. For best results, freeze them overnight.

The preparation time for Berry Coconut Ice Pops is approximately 10-15 minutes, plus freezing time. This recipe makes about 6-8 ice pops, depending on the size of your molds. Once frozen, these ice pops are ready to enjoy whenever you need a refreshing and healthy treat. They are perfect for kids and adults alike, providing a nutritious alternative to sugar-laden store-bought popsicles.

These Berry Coconut Ice Pops are a wonderful way to enjoy a sweet treat while still adhering to a Candida-friendly diet. The combination of antioxidant-rich berries and creamy coconut milk creates a delicious and satisfying dessert that supports your health and well-being. Enjoy them on a hot summer day or anytime you crave a cool, fruity snack!

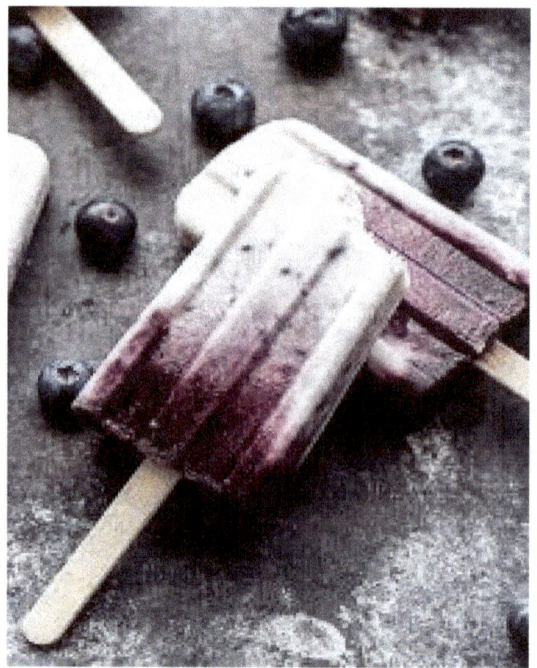

Berry Coconut Ice Pops

CANDIDA OVERGROWTH TREATMENT

INDULGENT SNACK IDEAS

■ Cacao Energy Balls

Cacao Energy Balls are a snack that combines the rich flavor of cacao with the natural sweetness of dates and the satisfying crunch of nuts and seeds. These bite-sized treats are perfect for a quick energy boost, making them ideal for busy days or as a pre- or post-workout snack. Cacao Energy Balls are packed with nutrients from various food classes, including carbohydrates from dates, healthy fats from nuts and seeds, and protein from both nuts and seeds. Additionally, they provide a dose of antioxidants from cacao, making them a well-rounded and healthful treat.

Ingredients:
To make Cacao Energy Balls, you will need:
i. Medjool dates: 1 cup, pitted
ii. Raw almonds: 1/2 cup
iii. Raw cashews: 1/2 cup
iv. Cacao powder: 1/4 cup
v. Chia seeds: 2 tablespoons
vi. Flaxseeds: 2 tablespoons, ground
vii. Coconut oil: 2 tablespoons, melted
viii. Vanilla extract: 1 teaspoon
ix. Sea salt: a pinch

x. Unsweetened shredded coconut: 1/4 cup (optional, for rolling)

Cooking Methods:
- ➢ **Prepare the Dates:** If the dates are a bit dry, soak them in warm water for about 10 minutes to soften. This will make them easier to blend. After soaking, drain the dates well.
- ➢ **Blend the Nuts:** In a food processor, pulse the raw almonds and cashews until they are finely ground. Be careful not to over-process, as you want a slightly coarse texture.
- ➢ **Combine Ingredients:** Add the pitted dates, cacao powder, chia seeds, ground flaxseeds, melted coconut oil, vanilla extract, and a pinch of sea salt to the food processor. Blend everything together until the mixture becomes smooth and sticky. If the mixture is too dry, you can add a small amount of water, one teaspoon at a time, until the desired consistency is reached.
- ➢ **Form the Balls:** Using your hands, scoop out small portions of the mixture and roll them into bite-sized balls. If desired, roll each ball in unsweetened shredded coconut for an extra layer of flavor and texture.

Making Cacao Energy Balls is a quick and easy process, typically taking about 20 minutes from start to finish. This recipe yields approximately 20-24 energy balls, depending on the size you make them. These energy balls can be stored in an airtight container in the refrigerator for up to two weeks, making them a convenient and long-lasting snack option. Perfect for when you need a quick, nutritious boost, Cacao Energy Balls are a tasty and healthful way to satisfy your sweet tooth while providing essential nutrients from whole food ingredients. Enjoy them as a guilt-free treat anytime you need a burst of energy!

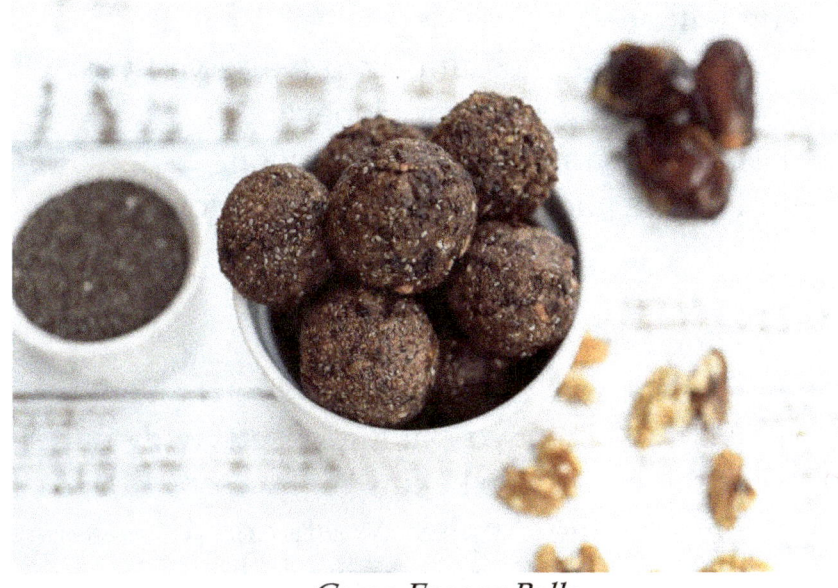

Cacao Energy Balls

■ Baked Apple Chips With Cinnamon

Baked Apple Chips with Cinnamon perfectly combines the natural sweetness of apples with the warm, comforting spice of cinnamon. This snack falls into the fruit category and provides essential nutrients such as dietary fiber, vitamins (particularly vitamin C), and antioxidants. Apples are known for their high fiber content, which supports digestive health, while cinnamon adds not only flavor but also potential anti-inflammatory benefits. These chips are a fantastic alternative to sugary snacks and are easy to make at home.

Ingredients:

To make Baked Apple Chips with Cinnamon, you will need:

i. Apples: 3-4 medium-sized (variety of your choice, such as Fuji, Gala, or Honeycrisp)
ii. Ground cinnamon: 1-2 teaspoons
iii. Lemon juice: 1 tablespoon (optional, to prevent browning)

Cooking Methods:
- **Preheat the Oven**: Preheat your oven to 200°F (95°C). Line two baking sheets with parchment paper or silicone baking mats.
- **Prepare the Apples:** Wash and dry the apples thoroughly. Using a sharp knife or a mandoline slicer, slice the apples as thinly as possible, ideally around 1/8 inch thick. Remove any seeds as you go. If you prefer, you can core the apples before slicing, but it's not necessary.
- **Optional Lemon Juice Step:** To prevent the apple slices from browning, you can lightly brush them with lemon juice. This step is optional but can help maintain the apples' natural color.

- ➢ **Season the Apples:** Arrange the apple slices in a single layer on the prepared baking sheets. Sprinkle the ground cinnamon evenly over the apple slices. You can adjust the amount of cinnamon to your taste preference.
- ➢ **Bake the Chips:** Place the baking sheets in the preheated oven. Bake the apple slices for about 1.5 to 2 hours, flipping them halfway through the baking time. The goal is to dry out the apples and make them crispy, so the exact time may vary depending on the thickness of the slices and your oven. Keep an eye on them to avoid burning.
- ➢ **Cool and Store:** Once the apple chips are crispy and lightly browned, remove them from the oven and let them cool completely on the baking sheets They will continue to crisp up as they cool. Store the cooled apple chips in an airtight container to keep them fresh and crunchy.

Baked Apple Chips with Cinnamon take about 1.5 to 2 hours to bake, plus additional time for cooling. This recipe yields approximately 4 servings, making it a great snack to share with family or friends. Each serving provides a nutritious, fiber-rich snack that satisfies sweet cravings without the added sugars or preservatives found in store-bought snacks. Enjoy these chips on their own, or use them as a crunchy topping for oatmeal, yogurt, or salads.

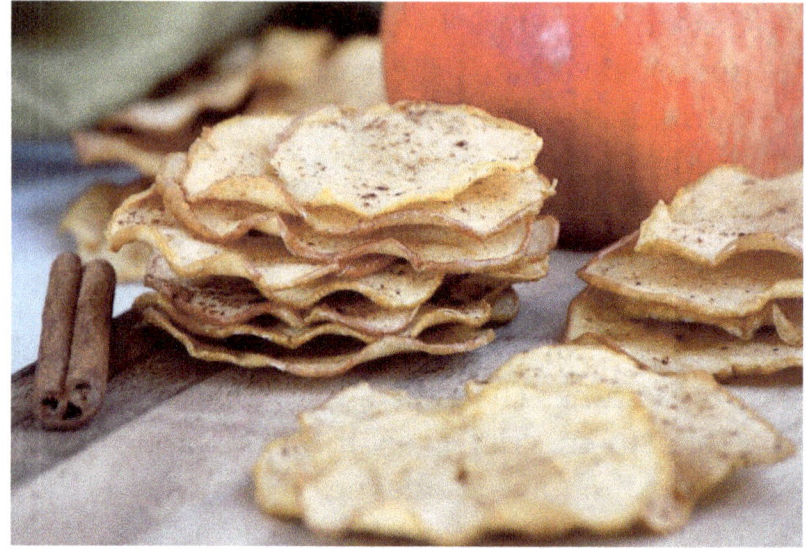
Baked Apple Chips With Cinnamon

▪ Chia Seed Coconut Pudding

Chia Seed Coconut Pudding combines the unique gelling properties of chia seeds with the creamy richness of coconut milk. This pudding is a fantastic addition to a Candida-friendly diet, offering a satisfying treat without the excessive sugars that can exacerbate Candida overgrowth. Chia seeds are classified as seeds, while coconut milk falls into the dairy alternatives category. Together, they provide a wealth of nutrients, including healthy fats, fiber, protein, and essential minerals like calcium and magnesium. This pudding is not only tasty but also incredibly nourishing, supporting overall health and well-being.

Ingredients:

To make Chia Seed Coconut Pudding, you will need:
i. Chia seeds: 1/4 cup
ii. Coconut milk: 1 cup (full-fat for a creamier texture, or light for a lower calorie option)
iii. Vanilla extract: 1 teaspoon
iv. Stevia or honey: 1-2 teaspoons (optional, for sweetness)
v. Fresh fruit or nuts for topping: such as berries, mango, almonds, or coconut flakes

Cooking Methods:

- **Mix the Ingredients:** In a medium-sized bowl, combine the chia seeds, coconut milk, vanilla extract, and sweetener (if using). Stir well to ensure that the chia seeds are evenly distributed and not clumping together.
- **Let it Sit:** Cover the bowl and refrigerate for at least 4 hours, or overnight for best results. During this time, the chia seeds will absorb the liquid and expand, creating a pudding-like consistency.
- **Stir Again:** After the pudding has set, give it another good stir to make sure the texture is smooth and the chia seeds are evenly distributed.
- **Serve:** Spoon the pudding into individual serving bowls or jars. Top with your choice of fresh fruit, nuts, or coconut flakes to add texture and flavor.

The Chia Seed Coconut Pudding requires minimal preparation time, typically around 5 minutes to mix the ingredients. The majority of the time is spent waiting for the pudding to set in the refrigerator, which takes at least 4 hours. This recipe makes about 2 servings, depending on portion sizes. Each serving is packed with nutrients, offering a good balance of healthy fats, fiber, and protein, making it a perfect snack or dessert that satisfies your cravings while supporting your Candida-friendly diet. Enjoy this creamy, nutritious pudding as a delightful way to nourish your body and treat your taste buds!

SUBSTITUTION GUIDE FOR CANDIDA-FRIENDLY INGREDIENTS

Candida-friendly diet can feel overwhelming, especially when it comes to finding suitable substitutes for common ingredients that you might be used to. But fear not! This guide is here to help you navigate through these changes with ease and confidence. By swapping out certain ingredients, you can enjoy delicious meals that support your health without compromising on flavor or variety. Let's explore some of the most common substitutions to help you on your Candida-friendly journey.

1. **Sweeteners:** One of the first things to address in a Candida-friendly diet is sugar. Refined sugars and high-fructose corn syrup are a big no-no, as they can feed Candida and exacerbate overgrowth. Here are some alternatives:
i. **Stevia:** A natural, zero-calorie sweetener derived from the leaves of the Stevia plant. It's much sweeter than sugar, so a little goes a long way.
ii. **Monk Fruit:** Another natural, calorie-free sweetener that doesn't affect blood sugar levels. Monk fruit extract can be used in baking, beverages, and more.
iii. **Erythritol:** A sugar alcohol that provides sweetness without the negative effects of sugar.

It's often used in combination with stevia or monk fruit to improve taste.

2. **Flours:** Traditional flours, especially those containing gluten, can be problematic for individuals managing Candida overgrowth. Here are some better options:
   i. **Almond Flour:** Made from finely ground almonds, this flour is low in carbs and high in healthy fats and protein. It's perfect for baking cakes, cookies, and bread.
   ii. **Coconut Flour:** This flour is made from dried coconut meat and is rich in fiber and healthy fats. It's very absorbent, so you'll need less of it compared to other flours.
   iii. **Chickpea Flour:** Also known as gram flour, chickpea flour is high in protein and fiber. It's great for savory dishes like fritters and flatbreads.

3. **Dairy:** Many people with Candida overgrowth find that reducing or eliminating dairy helps manage their symptoms. Here are some dairy-free alternatives:
   i. **Coconut Milk:** Rich and creamy, coconut milk is a versatile substitute for milk in cooking and baking. It's also great in smoothies and coffee.
   ii. **Almond Milk:** A lighter option that's perfect for cereal, baking, and beverages. Make sure to choose unsweetened versions.

iii. **Cashew Cream:** Made from blended cashews, this can be used as a substitute for cream in sauces and desserts. It has a rich, buttery flavor.

4. **Grains and Pasta:** Refined grains and pasta can spike blood sugar and feed Candida. Here are some healthier alternatives:
i. **Quinoa:** A high-protein seed that cooks up like a grain. It's great as a side dish, in salads, or even as a breakfast porridge.
ii. **Zucchini Noodles (Zoodles):** Made using a spiralizer, zoodles are a fantastic low-carb substitute for pasta. They're perfect in stir-fries, salads, and with your favorite sauces.
iii. **Cauliflower Rice:** Finely chopped cauliflower that mimics the texture of rice. It's an excellent low-carb alternative that can be used in a variety of dishes.

5. **Oils and Fats:** Healthy fats are essential in a Candida-friendly diet, but some oils can be inflammatory. Here are some better options:
i. **Coconut Oil:** Known for its antifungal properties, coconut oil is excellent for cooking and baking. It can also be used in smoothies and as a spread.
ii. **Olive Oil:** Rich in monounsaturated fats, olive oil is great for salad dressings, sautéing, and drizzling over cooked dishes.
iii. **Avocado Oil:** With a high smoke point, avocado oil is perfect for frying and roasting. It's also a good source of healthy fats.

6. **Condiments** Many store-bought condiments are loaded with sugar and preservatives. Here are some healthier options:
  i. **Homemade Salad Dressings:** Use olive oil, vinegar, and fresh herbs to create flavorful dressings without the added sugars and chemicals.
  ii. **Coconut Aminos:** A soy-free, gluten-free alternative to soy sauce made from the sap of coconut blossoms. It's lower in sodium and has a slightly sweet flavor.
  iii. **Mustard:** Most mustards are sugar-free and add a tangy kick to sandwiches, dressings, and marinades. Just be sure to check the label for added sugars.

7. **Snacks:** Finding Candida-friendly snacks can be tricky, but there are plenty of tasty options:
  i. **Nuts and Seeds:** Almonds, walnuts, sunflower seeds, and chia seeds are great for snacking and provide healthy fats and protein. Just be sure to choose raw or dry-roasted versions without added sugars.
  ii. **Vegetable Chips:** Kale chips, zucchini chips, and beet chips can be made at home or found in health food stores. They're a crunchy, satisfying alternative to traditional potato chips.
  iii. **Fresh Vegetables with Hummus:** Sliced cucumbers, bell peppers, and carrots dipped in

homemade hummus make a nutritious and filling snack.

8. **Beverages** Sugary drinks and caffeinated beverages can be detrimental to managing Candida. Here are some better alternatives:
i. **Herbal Teas:** Enjoy a variety of caffeine-free herbal teas like chamomile, peppermint, and ginger. They're soothing and beneficial for digestion.
ii. **Lemon Water**: A refreshing and alkalizing drink that's easy to make. Just add fresh lemon juice to water and enjoy.
iii. **Coconut Water:** Opt for unsweetened versions. Coconut water is hydrating and contains electrolytes, making it a great alternative to sugary sports drinks.

Transitioning to a Candida-friendly diet doesn't mean you have to give up your favorite foods. With these substitutions, you can continue to enjoy delicious and satisfying meals that support your health and well-being. Experiment with these alternatives, get creative in the kitchen, and most importantly, listen to your body. Making these changes can lead to improved health, more energy, and a better quality of life. Enjoy the journey to better health with these Candida-friendly substitutions!

CONCLUSION

Embarking on the journey of Candida-friendly cooking can feel like stepping into a new world of flavors, ingredients, and culinary techniques. It's more than just a dietary adjustment; it's a holistic approach to health that embraces the power of food to heal and nourish. As we conclude this book, I want to share some personal reflections and insights to inspire and guide you as you continue on this path.

Firstly, understanding Candida overgrowth and its impact on our bodies is the cornerstone of making informed food choices. By recognizing the symptoms and being aware of the foods that can exacerbate or alleviate these issues, you're already taking significant steps towards better health. This journey is about empowerment through knowledge, and I'm thrilled that we've been able to explore this together.

One of the most rewarding aspects of Candida-friendly cooking is discovering the vast array of delicious, nutrient-dense foods that support your well-being. From vibrant vegetables and lean proteins to wholesome grains and healthy fats, there's a rich variety of ingredients to experiment with. Recipes like Spinach and Avocado Soup, Beet and Arugula Salad with Citrus Dressing, and Chia Seed Coconut Pudding not only align with a

Candida-conscious diet but also showcase how tasty and satisfying these meals can be.

Cooking, in this context, transforms from a routine task into a form of self-care and creativity. It's about savoring the process of preparing meals that not only nourish your body but also delight your senses. The act of chopping fresh vegetables, blending a creamy smoothie, or roasting beets becomes a mindful practice, a way to connect with the food you eat and appreciate its role in your health journey.

Moreover, Candida-friendly cooking encourages us to think about balance and moderation. It's not about strict restrictions or feeling deprived. Instead, it's about making thoughtful choices that promote harmony within our bodies. By incorporating antifungal foods like garlic, onions, and coconut oil, and embracing probiotic-rich options like yogurt and kefir, we create an environment that supports healthy gut flora and overall wellness.

Another important aspect is the adaptability and flexibility of this approach. Life is dynamic, and so are our dietary needs. Whether you're cooking for yourself, your family, or hosting friends, Candida-friendly recipes can be adapted to suit various preferences and occasions. This versatility ensures that your meals are both enjoyable and healthful, without feeling like a burden.

It's also essential to acknowledge that the journey to managing Candida overgrowth is unique for everyone. There will be times of trial and error, moments of doubt, and days when sticking to your dietary plan feels challenging. But remember, every small step you take towards healthier eating habits is a victory. Celebrate your progress, no matter how minor it may seem, and be kind to yourself through the process.

In closing, I hope this book has provided you with the tools, recipes, and inspiration to embrace Candida-friendly cooking with confidence and enthusiasm. The goal is not just to manage Candida overgrowth, but to foster a deeper connection with the food you eat and its impact on your health. Cooking can be a joyful, empowering, and transformative experience, and I am honored to have shared this journey with you.

Here's to your continued health and happiness, and to the many delicious meals that lie ahead. May your kitchen be filled with the vibrant colors, enticing aromas, and nourishing flavors of Candida-friendly foods, and may you enjoy every bite on this path to wellness. Happy cooking!

www.ingramcontent.com/pod-product-compliance
Lightning Source LLC
Chambersburg PA
CBHW071936210526
45479CB00002B/706